U0251198

教育部、国家语委重大文化工程
"中华思想文化术语传播工程"成果
国家社科基金重大项目
"中国核心术语国际影响力研究"（项目号：21&ZD158）成果

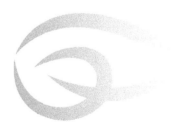

中华思想文化术语传播工程

Key Concepts in
Chinese Thought and Culture

邢玉瑞 编著

吴青 李晓莉 译

# 中医文化

# 关键词

## 汉英对照

## -3-

# Key Concepts in
# Traditional Chinese Medicine III

## (Chinese-English)

外语教学与研究出版社
FOREIGN LANGUAGE TEACHING AND RESEARCH PRESS
北京 BEIJING

**图书在版编目 (CIP) 数据**

中医文化关键词. 3：汉英对照 / 邢玉瑞编著 ；吴青，李晓莉译. -- 北京：外语教学与研究出版社，2024.5
ISBN 978-7-5213-5264-1

I. ①中… II. ①邢… ②吴… ③李… III. ①中国医药学－名词术语－汉、英 IV. ①R2-61

中国国家版本馆 CIP 数据核字 (2024) 第 106902 号

出 版 人　王　芳
责任编辑　钱垂君
责任校对　牛茜茜
封面设计　李　高　彩奇风
版式设计　XXL Studio
出版发行　外语教学与研究出版社
社　　址　北京市西三环北路 19 号（100089）
网　　址　https://www.fltrp.com
印　　刷　河北虎彩印刷有限公司
开　　本　710×1000　1/16
印　　张　17
字　　数　323 千字
版　　次　2024 年 5 月第 1 版
印　　次　2024 年 5 月第 1 次印刷
书　　号　ISBN 978-7-5213-5264-1
定　　价　78.00 元

如有图书采购需求，图书内容或印刷装订等问题，侵权、盗版书籍等线索，请拨打以下电话或关注官方服务号：
客服电话：400 898 7008
官方服务号：微信搜索并关注公众号"外研社官方服务号"
外研社购书网址：https://fltrp.tmall.com

物料号：352640001

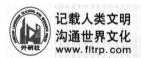

# 编写说明

　　《中医文化关键词 3》是中华思想文化术语之"中医文化关键词"主题系列的第三本。前两辑即《中医文化关键词》（2018 年，111 条）和《中医文化关键词 2》（2021 年，110 条），对精选的 221 条中医思想文化基本术语（主要围绕精、气、阴阳理论、五行、藏象、经络、病因病机和治法治则相关的概念）进行了阐释。本辑在前两册的基础上，增加了更具中医临床特色和文化特色的词汇，包括 100 个关键词、索引、参考书目和中国历史年代简表。翻译本辑时，使用的参考文献包括了 2022 年世界卫生组织（WHO）最新发布的《世界卫生组织中医药术语国际标准》。

　　本辑中每个关键词词条的内容，包含拼音、中文、英文、中文解释、英文解释、曾经译法（2000 年及之前出版作品中的翻译）、现行译法（2000 年后出版作品中的翻译）、推荐译法、翻译说明以及引例。读者通过阅读，不仅能够了解关键词的中文含义以及英文解释，还能够通过比较曾经译法和现行译法，结合翻译说明，了解中医翻译研究近 40 年来的发展变化。同时，引例可以帮助读者了解这些关键词在中医典籍中的具体应用。本辑采用中英文对照体例，对想要学习、了解和借鉴中医文化内涵的国内外读者大有裨益，也为中医药英译、中华文化传播与国际交流以及中医文献研究提供了宝贵的素材。

　　本辑在编写时仍然采用了与前两辑保持一致的基本原则，"曾经译法"和"现行译法"中的表述均引自书后所列的 35 条参考文献，单词拼写、大小写形式、括弧、连字符等语言、语法形式均保持原状。对于所引译文中显而易见的语法和语言错误，采用了括号加注或翻译说明的方式做了简要说明。需要说明的是，从 2018 年 5 月《中医文化关键词》出版至今已六年，期间中医药术语国际标准及其相关研究又有了一定的发展，故而本辑译者对书中出现的《黄帝内经》《灵枢》《神农本草经》等经典古籍的英译做了更新，将《黄帝内经》英译为 *Huangdi's Inner Canon of Medicine*、《灵枢》英译为 *Miraculous Pivot*、《神农本草经》英译为 *Shennong's Classic of Materia Medica*。此外，本辑涉及较多之前未被纳入《世界卫生组织中医药术语国际标准》等资料的语汇，故译者提出"推荐译法"，以供学界进一步研究确定。

# Note to Readers

*Key Concepts in Traditional Chinese Medicine III* is the third book of the series of *Key Concepts in Traditional Chinese Medicine*, which is under the national project of "Key Concepts in Chinese Thought and Culture." The first two of the series, *Key Concepts in Traditional Chinese Medicine* (published in 2018, containing 111 terms) and *Key Concepts in Traditional Chinese Medicine II* (published in 2021, containing 110 terms), have included 221 basic terms concerning the thoughts and culture of traditional Chinese medicine (TCM). They are mainly related to essence, qi, the theory of yin and yang, five elements, visceral manifestation, meridians, etiology, pathogenesis, and treatment principles and methods. *Key Concepts in Traditional Chinese Medicine III* includes another 100 key concepts with distinctive TCM clinical and cultural characteristics. A list of concepts, index, reference books, and a brief chronology of Chinese history are placed at the very end of the book. The references include the *WHO International Standard Terminologies on Traditional Chinese Medicine* issued in 2022.

Each listed concept is provided with mandarin pronunciation in pinyin, simplified Chinese characters, English translation, definitions in both Chinese and English, previous translation of the key concept (found in publications in and before 2000), current translation of the key concept (found in publications after 2000), recommended translation of the key concept, explanatory notes as well as citations from TCM classics in both Chinese and English. It is expected that readers not only understand the Chinese meaning and English translation of the key concepts but also gain a deeper understanding of the progress made over a period of 40 years in the translation studies of TCM key concepts by comparing their "previous translation" with their "current translation" in combination with the "explanatory notes." In addition, readers can gain an insight into the specific application of the included key concepts by referring to their corresponding citations. Being bilingual, this book can be a helpful resource to the readers at home and abroad who want to learn, understand, and draw on the fundamental concepts in TCM. It may serve as valuable reference material for the English translation of TCM texts, the international communication of Chinese culture, and the research of TCM literature.

The principle of consistency was still followed in this book. The English expressions in "previous translation" and "current translation" have been cited from 35 references listed at the end of the book, without changes in either language or grammar, i.e., spelling form, capitalization, use of brackets, and hyphens. Nevertheless, notes are either given in brackets or in "explanatory notes" for those that are obviously erroneous. It should be noted that the international standard terminologies on TCM have been updated and their research has been advanced since the publication of *Key Concepts in Traditional Chinese Medicine* in May, 2018. Therefore, slight changes are made on the translations of some ancient book names such as *Huangdi Neijing*《黄帝内经》, *Ling Shu*《灵枢》 and *Shennong Bencao Jing*《神农本草经》. The first is translated into *Huangdi's Inner Canon of Medicine*, the second, *Miraculous Pivot*, and the third, *Shennong's Classic of Materia Medica*. Besides, "recommended translation" is provided for further research since many key concepts in this book are not previously studied or included in the texts such as *WHO International Standard Terminologies on Traditional Chinese Medicine*.

# 前　言

中医是中国医药学的简称，是中国特有的一门与天文、地理和人文密切交融的古典医学体系。中医以中国的传统文化、古典哲学和人文思想为理论基础，融合诸子之学和百家之论，综合自然科学和社会科学的理论与实践，构建了独具特色的理论体系、思辨模式和诊疗方法。中医重视人与自然的和谐共处，强调文化传承的一以贯之，提倡人与社会的和谐发展，为各地医药的创建、文化的传播和文明的发展开辟了广阔的路径。这正如2016 年国务院颁布的《中国的中医药》白皮书对中医的文化定位，中医是"中华文明的杰出代表"，"对世界文明进步产生了积极影响"，"实现了自然科学与人文科学的融合和统一"，"蕴含了中华民族深邃的哲学思想"。

中医是目前世界上历史最为悠久、文化最为深厚、体系最为完整、疗效最为显著、应用最为广泛、发展最为迅速的一门传统医学体系。早在先秦时期，中医已经逐步传入朝鲜等周边地区。汉唐时期，中医已经传入日本、东南亚地区。18 世纪之后，中医逐步传入欧洲并在 19 世纪中期得到了较为广泛的传播。20 世纪 70 年代之后，随着针刺麻醉术的研制成功，中医很快传遍全球，为世界医药的发展，为各国民众的健康，为中华文化的传播做出了巨大的贡献。由于理法先进、文化深厚、方药自然、疗效神奇，中医这门古老的医学体系虽历经数千年而始终昌盛不衰，为中华民族的繁衍、为中华文明的发展、为中华文化的传播开辟了独特的蹊径。

中医的四大经典——即《黄帝内经》《难经》《神农本草经》《伤寒杂病论》——不仅代表着中医最为核心的理论和方法，而且还代表着中华文化最为核心的思想和精神，特别是《黄帝内经》，几乎涉及中国古代自然科学、社会科学和语言文化等各个方面。其在世界各地的传播已经成为中国文化走向世界的康庄大道。阴（yin）、阳（yang）、气（qi）等中国文化重要概念的音译形式已经成为西方语言中的通用语，这就是中医为中国文化走出去做出的一大贡献，为中国文化走出去奠定了坚实的语言基础。

中国文化要西传，要走向世界，自然需要有一个各国学术领域、文化领域和民间人士所关注的方面，借以引导各界人士关注中国文化。汉唐时期西域佛界人士千里迢迢到中原地区宣扬佛教，明清时期西方传教士远渡重洋到中国传播基督教，医药一直是他们凝聚人心和人力的一个重要的路径。作为中国传统文化不可分割的一个重要组成部分，中医对于推进中国文化走向世界，不仅是凝聚异国他乡人心和人力的一个重要渠道，而且还是直接传播和传扬中国传统文化的一个重要桥梁。任何一位想要学习、了解和借鉴中医理法方药的外国人士，首先必须要学习和掌握阴阳学说、五行学说和精气学说等中国传统文化的基本理论和思想，这已经成为国际间的一个共识。

由此可见，要使中国文化全面、系统地走向世界并为世界各国越来越多人士心诚意正地理解和接受，中医的对外传播无疑是一个最为理想而独特的坚实桥梁。

李照国，2018

# Preface

TCM, short for traditional Chinese medicine, is a classical medical system with Chinese characteristics that are closely integrated with astronomy, geography, and humanities. Based on traditional Chinese culture, classical philosophy, and humanistic thoughts, TCM, in combination with the various schools of thought and their exponents during the period from pre-Qin times to the early years of the Han Dynasty as well as the theories and practice of natural sciences and social sciences, constitutes the unique theoretical system, way of thinking as well as diagnosis and treatment methods. TCM has a high regard for the harmonious coexistence of man and nature. It emphasizes consistent cultural inheritance, advocates the harmonious development between man and society, and opens broad prospects for local medicine development, cultural dissemination and the progress of human civilization. As promulgated in the white paper "Traditional Chinese Medicine in China" by the State Council in 2016, TCM is "a representative feature of Chinese civilization," which "produces a positive impact on the progress of human civilization," "represents a combination of natural sciences and humanities," and "embraces profound philosophical ideas of the Chinese nation."

TCM is at the present time the most comprehensive and the most widely used traditional medical system in the world with the longest history, the most profound culture, the most distinctive effects, and the fastest development. Early in the pre-Qin period, TCM had been gradually introduced into the neighboring areas such as the Korean Peninsula. During the Han and Tang dynasties, it had been brought into Japan and Southeast Asia. After the eighteenth century, TCM was introduced into Europe and it gained wide dissemination in the mid-nineteenth century. After the 1970s, TCM quickly spread all over the world along with the success of acupuncture anesthesia, contributing substantially to the development of world medicine, the wellbeing of all nations and the dissemination of Chinese culture. Due to its advanced theory, profound cultural basis, natural therapy, and remarkable effectiveness, TCM has survived and prospered throughout the ages. It has blazed a unique path for the prosperity of the Chinese nation, the development of Chinese civilization, and the spread of Chinese culture.

Four TCM classics—*Huangdi's Inner Canon of Medicine*, *Canon of Difficult Issues*, *Shennong's Classic of Materia Medica*, and *Treatise on Cold*

*Damage and Miscellaneous Diseases*—not only represent the core of TCM theory and method but also contain the essence of thought and spirit in Chinese culture, among which *Huangdi's Inner Canon of Medicine* is the landmark. It involves almost every aspect of natural sciences, social sciences as well as language and culture in ancient China. Its worldwide spread has become a great way for Chinese culture to go global. The transliteration of important concepts of Chinese culture such as yin, yang, and qi has been adopted in Western languages. This is a great contribution made by TCM to the "going out" of Chinese culture, and it has laid a solid language foundation for Chinese culture to go global.

Chinese culture is going to spread to the West, to the world. Naturally, there is a need for attention from various academic, cultural, and civil sectors. In the Han and Tang dynasties, the Buddhists in Xiyu (the Western Regions) travelled all the way to the Central Plains to promote Buddhism whereas in the Ming and Qing dynasties Western missionaries worked their way to China to spread Christianity. In both cases, medicine has been an important means to rally public support. As an integral part of traditional Chinese culture, TCM not only plays an important role in rallying foreign support to stimulate Chinese culture to go global but also serves as a bridge to disseminate and promote traditional Chinese culture directly. It is an international consensus that anyone desiring to learn, understand, and draw on TCM theories, methods, formulas, and herbs shall first of all learn and acquire the basic theories and thoughts of traditional Chinese culture, for example, the theory of yin and yang, the theory of five elements, and the theory of essence and qi.

It can be seen that the international communication of TCM is undoubtedly an ideal, unique, and solid approach if Chinese culture is to go global in a comprehensive and systematic manner and to gain the heartfelt understanding and acceptance from the people worldwide.

Li Zhaoguo, 2018

# 目 录
**Contents**

yī yì tóngyuán

# 医易同源

Medicine and *Yi* Studies Have a Common Origin.

　　医易同源是指医理与易理同源于事物的阴阳变化。《周易》系统包括《易经》《易传》以及始于汉代的研究《周易》经、传的易学。易学阐述事物阴阳动静变化的道理，中医学研究、阐明人体阴阳盛衰消长的机制，两者在认识论和方法论上有相通之处。综观古今医易关系的研究，有医易同源、会通、两分等不同见解。从发生学角度而言，《周易》与中医理论同源于巫术以及先秦时代儒家、道家、阴阳诸家思想及其思维方式；就科学从自然哲学的分化及《易经》之后至隋唐间中医学的发展而言，医与易主要呈现为两分的状态；中医理论的建构及隋唐以后中医学的发展，又借用了易学的哲学原理、范畴及思维方式，有些医家将易学象数推演模式引入中医学，在医学界形成了以易理解释医理的流派，医学因而成为象数之学的分支。

The term means that the principles of medical science and those of *Yi* (changes) studies are derived from the changes of yin and yang qualities of things. The system of *The Book of Changes* includes *The Classic Text* (*Yi Jing* or *I Ching*), *The Commentaries* (*Yi Zhuan*), and the *Yi* studies since the Han Dynasty. Traditional Chinese medicine (TCM) and *Yi* studies are similar in epistemology and methodology. The former expounds the waxing and waning of yin and yang in the human body, whereas the latter discloses the movement and stillness of yin and yang of myriad things. In view of the studies throughout history on the relationship between medicine and *Yi* studies, three different opinions are found: they are of the same origin; they are separate theories; they merge together. In terms of the genesis of *The Book of Changes* and TCM theories, both medicine and *Yi* studies originated from ancient witchcraft as well as the thoughts and modes of thinking of Confucianism, Daoism, and various yin-yang schools in the pre-Qin period. In terms of the separation of science from natural philosophy and the development of TCM from the period of *The Book of Changes* to the Sui and Tang dynasties, medicine and *Yi* studies are largely divided. In the formulation of TCM theories and the development of TCM after the Sui and Tang dynasties, the philosophical principles, categories, and ways of thinking of *Yi* studies are found present. Some medical scholars incorporated the inferential model of emblems and numbers into TCM, forming a school of interpreting medical theory by employing the principles of *Yi* studies. Thus, TCM became part of the science of emblems and numbers.

【曾经译法】无

【现行译法】无

【推荐译法】Medicine and *Yi* studies have a common origin.

【翻译说明】"医易同源"指医学和易学的理论依据和哲学原理相通，两者同源于事物的阴阳变化，故译为 Medicine and *Yi* studies have a common origin。

引例 Citation:

◎《易》者，易也，具阴阳动静之妙；医者，意也，合阴阳消长之机。虽阴阳已备于《内经》，而变化莫大于《周易》，故曰天人一理者，一此阴阳也；医易同原者，同此变化也。(《类经附翼·医易义》)

（《易》即变易，它具有阴阳动静的玄妙；医学乃是以意推理之事，它包藏着阴阳变化的关键。虽然阴阳理论在《黄帝内经》中的论述已经很完备，但对于变化的理论没有什么比《周易》概括还大的。所以说天人同一道理，就是同一阴阳；医易同一本源，就是同于阴阳变化。）

*Yi* means changes, containing the movement and stillness of yin and yang. Medicine is a matter of inference and reasoning based on intuitive understanding, which contains the key to the changes of yin and yang. The yin-yang theory is fully discussed in *Huangdi's Inner Canon of Medicine*, whereas the theory of changes is largely summarized in *The Book of Changes*. The heaven-human oneness means the unity of yin and yang. A common origin of medicine and *Yi* studies means both are derived from the changes of yin and yang. (*Appendices to the Classified Classics*) yào shí tóngyuán

# 药食同源

Medicine and Food Have a Common Origin.

药食同源指中医学所使用的药物与食物均源自植物或动物等。人们在生活实践中发现了各种食物和药物的性味、功效，认识到许多食物可以药用，许多药物也可以食用，如粳米、赤小豆、山楂、乌梅、核桃、饴糖、小茴香、姜、蜂蜜、枸杞、山药等，很难界定究竟是药物还是食物，因而成为药食两用之品。药食同源的理论渊源可追溯到上古时期，西汉刘安《淮南子·修务训》、唐代孙思邈《千金要方·食治》和清代黄宫绣的《本草求真》卷九均提到食物具有与药物类似的作用，提示在治疗疾病时，某些情况下可考虑首选食物进行治疗。

The term means that both Chinese medicines and food are derived from plants or animal parts. The Chinese people have come to understand the property, taste, and effects of various foods and medicines in their everyday life and practice. They are aware that many foods can be used as medicines and many medicines can be used as foods, for example, japonica rice, red adzuki bean, hawthorn, black plum, walnut, maltose, cumin, ginger, honey, goji berry, and Chinese yam. Sometimes it is really a challenge to determine whether they are medicines or foods; therefore, they are the dual-use products for both medical and food purposes. The concept that medicine and food have a common origin can be traced back to the remote ages of China. It can be found in *Huainanzi* by Liu An of the Western Han Dynasty, *Essential Prescriptions Worth a Thousand Pieces of Gold* by Sun Simiao of the Tang Dynasty, and *An Inquiry into Materia Medica* by Huang Gongxiu of the Qing Dynasty. They all stated that food could provide people with similar effects of medicine, suggesting that food can be considered as the first choice for disease treatment in certain cases.

【曾经译法】无

【现行译法】无

【推荐译法】Medicine and food have a common origin.

【翻译说明】参照"医易同源"的译法，"药食同源"可译为 Medicine and food have a common origin。医学文献数据库 PubMed 刊载的多篇论文将"药食同源"译为 medicine food homology。译词 homology 常表示物质结构、关系等的同源性。根据语境，"药食同源"也可译为 medicine food homology。


引例 Citation:


◎ 食以养生，药以治病，并皆神农之事。先君国材公尚谓药食同源者以此。（《神农古本草经》）

（食物用来滋养生命，药物用来治疗疾病，这些都是神农时代的事了。已故的父亲国材曾说药食同源，即因为这个原因。）

Food is to nourish and maintain life, whereas medicine is to treat diseases. This has been the way since the time of Shennong. Hence, my late father Guocai once stated that medicine and food had a common origin. (*Shennong's Ancient Classic of Materia Medica*) zhìyīn zhìyáng

# 稚阴稚阳

Immature Yin and Yang

稚阴稚阳是中医学对小儿生理特点的认识，认为小儿在物质基础和生理功能上，都处于幼稚和不完善的阶段。其阳气初生，血气未充，经脉未盛，脏腑娇嫩，内脏精气未足，神气怯弱，防御外邪功能未固，阴精阳气皆属不足，这是小儿的生理特点。正由于此，在病理情况下，小儿易于感邪发病，且一旦发病，又传变迅速，易于变化，易虚易实，易寒易热。在治疗用药时，不但应守护柔弱之阴津，也当固密稚嫩之阳气，以令阴阳和谐。稚阴稚阳说的确立，使中医学从功能和物质的角度对小儿生理体质的认识趋向全面，有助于理解小儿疾病易虚易实、易寒易热的病理变化。治疗疾病时，同样情况下可考虑首选食物治疗。

The term describes the physiological characteristics of children from the perspective of traditional Chinese medicine (TCM). It means that children are immature and underdeveloped in terms of material basis and physiological function. Children tend to have insufficient yang qi and blood, not-yet-fully-developed blood vessels, delicate *zang-fu* organs, inadequate essential qi of the internal organs, and weak body defense. Their yin and yang are not sufficient for them to fend off invasion of external pathogenic factors. Hence, children are susceptible to pathogenic factors under pathological conditions, and their disease will transmit quickly and change fast once it occurs. Pediatric cases tend to present with signs not only of deficiency or excess, but also of cold or heat. Treatment therefore should focus on protecting their yin aspect and strengthening their yang qi to achieve yin-yang harmony. The concept of immature yin and yang provides a comprehensive picture of children's physiological characteristics from the perspectives of function and material basis in TCM. It is conducive to the understanding of pathological changes of children's diseases that are characterized by the likelihood of manifesting deficiency or excess patterns as well as cold or heat patterns. In the treatment of pediatric diseases, food can be considered as the first choice when it has the same effect as medicine.

【曾经译法】 young yang and young yin; tender yang and tender yin; premature yin and yang

【现行译法】 young yin and young yang; young yang and young yin; young yang and yin; premature yang and yin; immature yin and yang; premature yin and yang; immature yin-yang; tender yin, tender yang

【推荐译法】 immature yin and yang

【翻译说明】 "稚" 对应的译文有四种，包括 young（年轻的）、tender（温柔的；脆弱的；嫩的）、immature（幼稚的；发育未全的）和 premature（未成熟的；过早的；提前的）。"稚" 表示稚嫩、幼稚、不完善，因此 immature 较为恰当。


引例 Citations:


◎ 古称小儿纯阳，此丹灶家言，谓其未曾破身耳，非盛阳之谓。小儿稚阳未充，稚阴未长者也。（《温病条辨·解儿难》）

（古代称小儿是纯阳之体，这是古代炼丹术士的说法，意思是小儿还是童真之体，并不是指阳气偏盛。小儿的阴阳，都还没有达到成熟阶段。）

Children are considered pure yang in nature by ancient Chinese alchemists, meaning that they possess innocence and virginity, but not that their yang qi is excessive. The yin and yang of children are still growing, far from reaching maturity. (*Systematic Differentiation of Warm Diseases*)

◎ 小儿……稚阳未充，稚阴未长者也。稚阳未充，则肌肤疏薄，易于感触；稚阴未长，则脏腑柔嫩，易于传变，易于伤阴。（《医原·儿科论》）

（小儿……其阴阳都还没有达到成熟阶段。稚弱的阳气没有充盛，则肌肤疏松薄弱，容易感受外邪；稚弱的阴气没有旺盛，则脏腑柔嫩，疾病容易传变，容易损伤阴气。）

For children... their yin and yang are far from reaching maturity. When yang qi is not fully produced, their skin will be soft, loose, and weak, and children are thus prone to the invasion of external pathogenic factors. When yin qi is not yet fully generated, their *zang-fu* organs are tender, and diseases are likely to transmit and change, which in turn will readily impair yin qi. (*Bases of Medicine*) *gāoliáng*

# 膏粱

Rich Fare

膏粱，肥肉和细粮，泛指肥美的食物，也可代指富贵人家或生活奢靡的人。富贵者饮食甘美厚味，生活安逸少动，容易助湿生痰，形成痰湿体质。此类体质的人易患消渴、中风、眩晕、女性不孕等疾病，治疗应注意选用渗湿化痰的方药。

The term, meaning fat meat and fine grains, refers to fatty and delicious food in general. It also refers to rich and noble families or people living in luxury. The rich and noble people tend to eat rich-flavored foods and dishes, live a comfortable life with little activity, and are thus susceptible to producing phlegm, developing a phlegm-dampness constitution. People with this type of constitution are prone to diseases such as wasting and thirst disorders, stroke, vertigo, and female infertility. Treatment should focus on draining dampness and resolving phlegm.

【曾经译法】 fatty diet; fatty foods and delicious drinks; rich fatty diet; rich food; fat meat, fine grain, and strong flavors [rich food]; greasy diet

【现行译法】 greasy food; greasy diet; Fatty and Sweet Food; rich and flavored food; greasy and surfeit flavour; rich fatty diet; greasy diet/rich diet; rich food; Rich and fatty diet; rich and heavy flavored food; fatty foods and delicious drinks; fat rich food

【推荐译法】 rich fare

【翻译说明】 综观以往译法，"膏粱"多译为 greasy，fatty 或 rich。前两个词侧重表示"油腻的""富含脂肪的"，第三个词可表示"油腻的；高热量的；丰富的"。译词 fare 表示饮食，为书面语。

因"膏粱"泛指肥美的食物，建议采用 rich fare 翻译本词条，概念相对宽泛。

◎ 贵贱尊卑，劳逸有异，膏粱藜藿，气质不同，故当度民君卿，分别上下以为诊。(《类经·脉色类》)

（富贵与贫贱，地位高与下，劳作与安逸不同，肥美之食与粗疏的饭菜，人的气质有别。因此，必须考虑患者是普通百姓还是达官贵人，区分患者地位的高低再进行诊治。）

Rich, high-status people are different from poor, low-status ones in terms of diet, labor, and leisure commitments. Rich fare and lowly fare nurture different temperaments. Therefore, for disease diagnosis and treatment, it is necessary to consider whether the patients are dignitaries or civilians and whether their social status is high or low. (*Classified Classics*)

◎ 膏粱自奉者脏腑恒娇，藜藿苟充者脏腑恒固。(《医宗必读·富贵贫贱治病有别论》)

（日常生活享用肥美之食者，脏腑常娇弱；随便用粗疏饭菜充腹者，脏腑常坚固。）

Those who are indulged in rich fare in daily life tend to have delicate *zang-fu* organs. Those who fill their bellies with lowly fare tend to have strong internal organs. (*Required Readings from the Medical Ancestors*) líhuò

# 藜藿

Lowly Fare

藜藿，指粗疏的饭菜，也可代指贫贱的人。贫贱的人饮食粗疏，劳作过度，易致气血不足或阴精亏少，形成气、血、阴、阳不足等虚性体质。此类体质的人易患感冒、汗出、咳嗽、泄泻、痰饮、便秘、内热等疾病，治疗当注意调补气血阴阳。

The term refers to coarse and simple food. It also refers to poor low-status people. Poor low-status people usually eat poorly and work excessively hard, which may lead to insufficiency of qi and blood or yin deficiency, and thus develop deficiency of qi, blood, yin, and yang. People with deficiency-type constitutions are prone to colds, sweating, cough, diarrhea, phlegm, constipation, internal heat, and other disorders. Attention should be given to regulating and replenishing qi, blood, yin, and yang.

【曾经译法】无

【现行译法】无

【推荐译法】lowly fare

【翻译说明】"藜藿"指粗疏的饭菜，与"膏粱"（rich fare）相对，可译为 lowly fare。

引例 Citations:

◎ 故膏粱之人多肥甘之渴、石药之渴，藜藿奔走之人多燥热之渴，二者虽殊，其实一也。（《儒门事亲》卷三）

（因此，富贵之人多因过食肥甘厚味之品或矿物类药物而患消渴，贫贱劳作之人多因燥热而成消渴，二者原因不同，但发为消渴则相同。）

Therefore, rich and noble people tend to have wasting and thirst disorders due to excessive intake of fatty and rich-flavored food or mineral drugs, whereas poor laborers who fill their bellies with lowly fare tend to have wasting and thirst disorders due to dryness and heat. Though the causes are different, both have the same disease. (*Confucians' Duties to Their Parents*)

◎ 医藜藿病，忌大温补，宜兼解肌润燥。(《王氏医存·贫富劳佚证治不同》)

（诊治贫贱之人的疾病，切忌过于温补，应该兼以解除肌表之邪并润燥。）

Overuse of warming therapy and tonics should be avoided in treating poor low-status patients. Instead, the treatment should focus on removing pathogenic factors from superficies and moistening dryness. (*Wang's Surviving Medicine*)

# 禀赋

Natural Endowment; Constitution

禀赋，又称先天禀赋，指个体在先天遗传的基础上、胎孕期间内外环境的影响下，所表现出的形态结构、生理功能、心理状态等方面综合的、相对稳定的特征。先天禀赋是人体体质形成的基础，是人体体质强弱的前提条件，它决定着人的寿夭、生命的质量以及个体受病与否和对于一些疾病的易感性。禀赋具有先天性、个体性、地域性、种族性和可调性，先天性是其最根本的特征。其各个特征之间相互联系，并且均受后天影响。禀赋的影响因素很多，遗传和环境是影响禀赋的主要因素，环境包括孕妇体内的小环境和体外的大生态环境，以及社会环境和心境。

The term is also known as congenital endowment or constitution. It refers to the overall and relatively constant characteristics of an individual's physical, physiological, and mental makeup as a result of heredity and effect of internal and external factors on prenatal development. It forms the basis of constitution and predefines physical strength. It also affects one's life span, quality of life, whether one acquires a disease, and whether one is vulnerable to certain diseases. Endowment is congenital, and is the most fundamental feature. It varies among people, across regions and ethnic groups, and could be regulated. These characteristics are interrelated. All are affected by a number of factors, among which heredity and environment play an important role. The latter includes the micro environment inside a pregnant woman's body and the macro, external, ecological, and social environment as well as individual mindset.

【曾经译法】无

【现行译法】natural endowment; constitution

【推荐译法】natural endowment; constitution

【翻译说明】根据上下文语境，可译为 natural endowment 或 constitution。

引例 Citations:

◎ 夫禀赋为胎元之本，精气之受于父母者是也。(《类经·疾病类》)

（先天禀赋是母体中培育胎儿生长发育的元气的根本，此乃禀受于父母的精气。）

Natural endowment is the foundation of primordial qi rooted in the kidney of the mother to ensure fetal growth and development. It is derived from the essential qi of parents. (*Classified Classics*)

◎ 其禀赋也，体有刚柔，脉有强弱，气有多寡，血有盛衰，皆一定而不易也。(《圣济经·原化篇》)

（由于先天禀赋，人体有刚有柔，脉象有强有弱，气有多有少，血有盛有衰，这些都是固定而不会变化的。）

Natural endowment determines whether the body is rigid or flexible, the pulse is strong or weak, qi is more or less, and blood is abundant or deficient. It is unlikely to change. (*Classic of Sacred Benevolence*) chóng yīn bì yáng

# 重阴必阳

Extreme Yin Transforms into Yang.

重阴必阳是中医学对于阴阳转化规律的一种认识。重，重叠、极之意。阴阳在一定条件下可以向对立面转化，阴阳转化的条件中医学称之为"重"或"极"，故曰"重阴必阳，重阳必阴""寒极生热，热极生寒"等。重阴必阳语出《素问·阴阳应象大论》："重阴必阳……冬伤于寒，春必病温"。因冬天本寒，又伤于寒，两寒相加是为重寒。同气相求，寒邪伤肾，如立即发病，可出现寒邪直中阴经之病；如未立即发病，则寒邪隐藏在身体的深位，等待春天阳气发越时，所受的寒邪外合阳邪外发而变发为温病，是受于阴而发于阳。

The term describes an understanding of mutual transformation between yin and yang in traditional Chinese medicine. *Chong* (重) means overlapping or extremity. Under certain circumstances, yin or yang will turn into its opposite. The condition for transformation is "overlapping" or "extremity." That is, "when yin develops to its extremity, it will transform into yang; when yang develops to its extremity, it will transform into yin." There are also such sayings as "extreme cold generates heat, and extreme heat generates cold." The expression, extreme yin transforming into yang, can be found in *Plain Conversation* ("Significant Discussions on Phenomena Corresponding to Yin and Yang"). It reads: "When yin develops to its extremity, it will transform into yang... If one is invaded by cold pathogen in winter, one will for sure develop warm diseases in spring." When one's health is damaged by cold pathogen in cold months, cold will double and develop to its extremity. Then the kidney (a yin organ) will be impaired because like attracts like. If there is immediate occurrence of the disease, it will be the result of cold pathogen directly attacking yin meridians. If not, cold pathogen will hide deep in the body and develop into warm diseases in spring as a result of cold pathogen mingling with yang pathogen when yang qi rises. The disease is characterized by invasion of yin pathogen, yet with yang manifestations.

【曾经译法】 overabundance of yin reverses to yang; inevitable transmutation of the superposed yin into yang; overabundance of yin transforming to yang; Extreme yin turns into yang; double yin becomes yang; yin in its extreme giving rise to yang; excessive yin leading to yang

【现行译法】 extreme yin turning into yang; overabundance of Yin transforming to Yang; extreme Yin giving rise to Yang; inevitable transmutation of the superposed yin into yang; extreme yin changing into yang; extreme yin leading to yang; Extreme yin transforming into yang

【推荐译法】 Extreme yin transforms into yang.

【翻译说明】 "重阴必阳"的"重"是"重叠，极"之意，译为 extreme（极度；极限）较妥，而非 overabundance（过剩，过多）或 superposed（叠放的）。"重阴必阳"表示阴阳在一定条件下可以向对立面转化。"转化"采用 transform，比 turn into, lead to, give rise to, change into 等更准确。译词 reverse 常用于表示"颠倒；撤销；交换位置；倒退行驶"等意思，与"转化"的意思相去甚远；译词 transmutation 多表示"变形；嬗变；衍变"。


引例 Citations:


◎ 然而物极则反，寒暑之变，重阳必阴，重阴必阳，阴证似阳，阳证似阴。（《活人书》卷四）

（但是物极必反，寒热的变化，阳气过盛一定转化为阴，阴气过盛一定转化为阳，或阴证疑似于阳证，阳证疑似于阴证。）

However, when a thing reaches its extremity, it reverses. In terms of mutual transformation of heat and cold, extreme yang transforms into yin, and extreme yin transforms into yang; or yin pattern looks like yang pattern and yang pattern looks like yin pattern. (*Book for Saving Lives*)

◎ 重阴必阳，重阳必阴，言阳极生阴，阴极生阳也。(《医门棒喝·伤寒论本旨》)

（阴气过盛一定转化为阳，阳气过盛一定转化为阴，是说阳极盛而变生为阴，阴极盛而变生为阳。）

Extreme yin transforms into yang, and extreme yang transforms into yin. In other words, when yin develops to its extremity, it will transform into yang; and when yang develops to its extremity, it will transform into yin. (*Medical Warnings*) chóng yáng bì yīn

# 重阳必阴

Extreme Yang Transforms into Yin.

重阳必阴，是中医学对于阴阳转化规律的一种认识。重阳必阴语出《素问·阴阳应象大论》，主要是从发病的角度阐述阴阳的转化关系，如"重阳必阴……春伤于风，夏生飧泄"。春本属阳，风为阳邪，气通肝胆。春伤于风，为重阳，若不立即发病，而留连于夏，脾经湿土当令，木邪来乘，而发为完谷不化的飧泄（阴证）。张介宾《类经·阴阳类》说："重者，重叠之义。谓当阴时而复感寒，阳时而复感热，或以天之热气伤人阳分，天之寒气伤人阴分，皆谓之重。盖阴阳之道，同气相求，故阳伤于阳，阴伤于阴。然而重阳必变为阴证，重阴必变为阳证。"

The term describes an understanding of mutual transformation between yin and yang in traditional Chinese medicine from the etiological viewpoint. It can be found in *Plain Conversation* ("Significant Discussions on Phenomena Corresponding to Yin and Yang"): "When yang develops to its extremity, it will transform into yin... If one is invaded by wind pathogen in spring, one will have diarrhea with undigested food in stools in summer." The spring season pertains to yang and wind is ascribed to yang pathogen. Its qi communicates with the liver and the gallbladder. If one is invaded by wind pathogen in spring, it amounts to extreme yang. If the pathogen does not readily incur disease but lingers on to the summer season (yang) when the spleen (earth) governs, the liver (wood) will over restrain the spleen, leading to diarrhea with undigested food (yin pattern) in summer. According to Zhang Jiebin's *Classified Classics*, "*Chong* (重) means overlapping, referring to the fact that one is invaded by cold (yin) in the season of yin and by heat (yang) in the season of yang, or one's yin aspect is affected by cold and one's yang aspect affected by heat. In terms of the law of yin and yang, like attracts like. Therefore, yang is damaged by yang; yin is damaged by yin. When yang develops to its extremity, it will transform into yin; when yin develops to its extremity, it will transform into yang."

【曾经译法】 overabundance of yang reverses to yin; inevitable transmutation of the superposed yang into yin; overabundance of yang transforming to yin; Extreme yang turns into yin; double yang becomes yin; yang in its extreme giving rise to yin; excessive yang leading to yin

【现行译法】 extreme yang turning into yin; overabundance of Yang transforming to Yin; extreme Yang giving rise to Yin; inevitable transmutation of the superposed yang into yin; extreme yang changing into yin; Extreme yang transforming into yin

【推荐译法】 Extreme yang transforms into yin.

【翻译说明】 "重阳必阴"的"重"是"重叠, 极"之意, 译为 extreme（极度; 极限）较妥, 而非 overabundance（过剩, 过多）或 superposed（叠放的）。"重阳必阴"表示阴阳在一定条件下可以向对立面转化。"转化"采用 transform, 比 turn into, lead to, give rise to, change into 等更准确。译词 reverse 常用于表示"颠倒; 撤销; 交换位置; 倒退行驶"等意思, 与"转化"的意思相去甚远; 译词 transmutation 多表示"变形; 嬗变; 衍变"。

引例 Citations:

◎ 此名阳证似阴也, 重阳必阴, 重阴必阳, 寒暑之变也。（《活人书》卷四）

（这个叫阳证疑似于阴证, 阳气过盛一定转化为阴, 阴气过盛一定转化为阳, 乃寒热之间的变化。）

It is called yang patterns looking like yin patterns. Extreme yang transforms into yin, and extreme yin transforms into yang. This is the transformation between cold and heat. (*Book for Saving Lives*)

◎ 经曰寒极生热，热极生寒，又曰重阴必阳，重阳必阴是也。(《读素问钞》卷下)

> (《内经》说寒极盛则变生热，热极盛则变生寒，又说阴气过盛一定转化为阳，阳气过盛一定转化为阴。)

*Huangdi's Inner Canon of Medicine* states that extreme cold generates heat, and extreme heat generates cold. It also states that extreme yin transforms into yang, and extreme yang transforms into yin. (*Notes Taken While Reading "Plain Conversation"*) guòyóu-bùjí

# 过犹不及

Too Much Is as Bad as Too Little.

过犹不及，指做事过了头，就如同做得不够一样，强调做事以适度为贵。这是中国传统文化"中庸""中和"观念的反映。中医学从这一哲学理念出发，提出了中和的健康观，失中的病因观，失和的疾病观以及求和、适中的养生与治疗观等。人体的健康乃是人体脏腑、气血、阴阳、形神以及人与环境之间关系的和谐。疾病乃是由于"生病起于过用"（《素问·经脉别论》），即对上述和谐状态的破坏，如《素问·调经论》云："血气不和，百病乃变化而生"。诊治疾病与养生以中和为最佳境界，治疗当"和"以所宜，令其条达，达到人与自然以及人体气血、阴阳、形神的有机和谐。

The term means exceeding is just as wrong as falling short of the line, and indicates that moderation is valued. It reflects the doctrine of "golden mean" and "balanced harmony" in traditional Chinese culture, based on which traditional Chinese medicine has put forward the following concepts: health is the balance between yin and yang; the cause of disease is the loss of balance; disease is disharmony; the goal of health preservation and treatment is to seek and restore harmony and moderation. Individual wellbeing can be defined as harmony among the *zang-fu* organs, qi and blood, yin and yang, body and spirit, as well as human and nature. Disease occurs when the above-mentioned harmonious relationships are disrupted by overuse (*Plain Conversation*, "Special Discussion on Meridians and Vessels"). For example, it is stated in *Plain Conversation* ("Discussion on the Regulation of Meridians") that "various diseases may arise if qi and blood are not in harmony." Balanced harmony is the primacy of diagnosis, treatment, and health cultivation. Treatment should focus on harmonization to achieve organic relationships of human and nature, qi and blood, yin and yang, as well as body and spirit.

【曾经译法】无

【现行译法】无

【推荐译法】 Too much is as bad as too little.

【翻译说明】 中华文化思想术语库也收录了"过犹不及"这一关键词，意思是事物超过一定的标准和没有达到标准同样不好。儒家以礼作为个人言语行事及其与天地万物关系的标准，并根据礼的要求判断言行的"过"或"不及"，故而翻译为 Going too far is as bad as falling short。在中医语境下，建议译为 Too much is as bad as too little。

引例 Citations:

◎ 六气之旨各居六十日有奇，以其时而化其气，过犹不及，病乃生焉，故察其盛衰而折之。(《校刻伤寒图歌活人指掌》卷一)

（六气各主时间为 60 天有余，按各自所主时段表现出不同的气候变化，太过犹如不及，会导致人体生病。因此，要观察六气的盛衰而进行调理。）

Each of the six qi governs a period of over 60 days respectively, presenting varied climatic characteristics accordingly. Too much is as bad as too little. Both may cause diseases. Therefore, it is necessary to regulate human body systems in accordance with the predominance or debilitation of the six qi. (*Corrected Verses of Cold Damage: A Simple Guide to Saving Lives*)

◎ 富贵之家过暖更十居八九，不知过犹不及也。(《救偏琐言》卷十)

（富贵人家过于温暖者更是十个中有八九个，不了解太过犹如不及之理。）

About 80-90% of wealthy families live in rooms that are too warm. They fail to perceive the concept that too much is as bad as too little. (*Notes on Treating Skin Eruptions*) bùtōng zé tòng

# 不通则痛

Where There Is Blockage, There Is Pain.

不通则痛，指气血运行不畅，阻滞于经络、脏腑等处可引起疼痛。如因外伤而致气滞血瘀，感受风、寒、湿邪而致经气痹阻，心脉瘀阻而致胸痹等，均可由不通而发生疼痛，故曰"不通则痛"。此为中医学对实证疼痛病机的概括，治疗当以通畅气血为法。

The term means that pain will occur as a result of unsmooth flow of qi or blood and their blockage in the meridians, collaterals, or *zang-fu* organs. For example, one may suffer from pain when there is qi stagnation and blood stasis caused by trauma, meridian-qi stagnation caused by invasion of wind, cold, or dampness, or chest-*bi* (impediment) caused by blockage of heart blood vessels. All these pains are attributed to blockage. The term summarizes the pathogenesis of excess pattern of pain. The goal of treatment is to unblock qi and blood.

【曾经译法】 when there is stoppage, there is pain

【现行译法】 stagnation leading to pain/obstruction resulting in pain; Obstruction Leads to Pain; pain due to stagnation of qi and blood

【推荐译法】 Where there is blockage, there is pain.

【翻译说明】 "不通则痛"指气血运行不畅，阻滞于经络、脏腑等处可引起疼痛。仿拟 Where there is a will, there is a way.（有志者事竟成）句子结构，可将"不通则痛"译为 Where there is blockage, there is pain。

引例 Citations:

◎ 寒为阴中之阴，乘于肌肉筋骨之间，营卫闭塞，筋骨拘挛，不通则痛，故为痛痹。(《医醇賸义》卷四)

（寒邪的属性为阴中之阴，侵袭肌肉筋骨之间，营卫之气闭塞不通，筋骨拘急挛缩，不通则导致疼痛，因此形成痛痹。）

Cold pathogen pertains to yin within yin, invading what lies in between muscles, tendons, and bones. As a result of stagnation in nutrient and defense qi, tendons and bones are constrained by contracture, leading to pain, and finally painful impediment. (*The Refined in Medicine Remembered*)

◎ 因其人卫气虚腠理不密，贼风乘虚而入客于经络，营卫不通则痛。(《针灸逢源》卷六)

（因为这个人卫气亏虚，腠理疏松，外邪乘虚侵入人体经络，营卫之气不通就疼痛。）

Because the patient has deficient defense aspect and loose muscular interstices, external pathogenic factors will invade their meridians by taking advantage of the weakness. Pain will occur when nutrient qi and defense qi are blocked. (*Effectiveness of Acupuncture and Moxibustion*) jiǔbìng rù luò

# 久病入络

Long-standing Disease Affects Collaterals.

久病入络，包括久痛入络，是清代著名医学家叶天士提出的诊治慢性病的思路之一。叶天士在大量临床实践中体会到，凡慢性疾患，都是病邪稽留的结果，最终必然伤及血络。病有新久，有在经在络、在气在血之分。疾病初期，邪气轻浅，多见于气分而在经。久则病邪渐渐深入，病位已深，多伤及血分而在络。对于慢性腹痛、胃脘痛、胁痛、疟疾、泄泻、便血、癥瘕等久治不愈的慢性疾病，叶天士按"久病入络"的思想进行辨证，运用通络法治疗，选方遣药除活血化瘀药物外，还常配伍辛散、温通、香窜之品以宣通气机，配虫类药搜风通络，取得了良好疗效。

The term, encompassing the concept of enduring pain affecting collaterals, offers a clue to the treatment of chronic diseases. It was proposed by Ye Tianshi, a distinguished physician of the Qing Dynasty. He concluded, based on his vast clinical practice, that chronic diseases were generally caused by the lingering pathogen that would eventually affect blood collaterals. The disease can be new or long-standing, affecting meridians, collaterals, qi, or blood. In the early stage of the disease, the pathogen affects superficially, mostly qi and meridians. After a prolonged period, the disease may go deeper, affecting blood and collaterals. For chronic abdominal pain, epigastric pain, hypochondriac pain, malaria, diarrhea, blood stool, abdominal mass, and other intractable chronic diseases, Ye Tianshi made pattern differentiation according to the concept of "long-standing disease affecting collaterals" and adopted the method of dredging collaterals. In addition to medicines for promoting blood circulation and removing blood stasis, he often incorporated pungent, warm, and aromatic ingredients into his prescriptions to promote qi activity, along with the use of insect-derived medicines to expel wind and dredge collaterals. Good clinical outcomes were usually obtained.

【曾经译法】无

【现行译法】collaterals affected in chronic diseases; chronic disease affecting
collaterals

【推荐译法】Long-standing disease affects collaterals.

【翻译说明】"久病"不宜翻译为 chronic disease（慢性病），根据上下文，
建议译为 long-standing disease。


引例 Citations:


◎ 所云初病在经，久痛入络，以经主气、络主血，则可知其治气治血之
当然也。（《临证指南医案·胃脘痛》）

（所说疾病初期在经脉，疼痛日久深入络脉，因经脉主气，络脉
主血，便可以知道治气、治血乃应当之事。）

In the early stage, disease affects meridians. If pain is prolonged, in-depth
collaterals will be affected. Since meridians govern qi and collaterals govern
blood, it is self-evident whether the focus of the treatment is to treat qi aspect or
blood aspect. (*Case Records: A Guide to Clinical Practice*)

◎ 初病在经，久病入络。（《类证治裁·内景综要》）

（疾病初期在经脉，疾病日久深入络脉。）

The disease affects meridians at its onset and will involve collaterals when it is
prolonged. (*Categorized Patterns with Clear-cut Treatments*)

qióng bì jí shèn

# 穷必及肾

Prolonged Morbidity Affects the Kidney.

穷必及肾，即久病必然影响到肾。中医学认为肾为先天之本，藏先天之精与后天之精，肾中精气是机体生命活动的根本，肾阴、肾阳均以肾精为其物质基础。生理情况下，肾接受五脏六腑的精气加以贮藏，各脏腑除在自身生理活动中消耗掉一定的精气外，剩余之精气输送并藏于肾中，故"肾为精之舍"。正因为如此，若其他脏腑受损导致阴阳失调时，一方面其他脏腑无精气归藏于肾，另一方面肾需输送精气到其他脏腑，以维持其最低限度的功能活动，日久必然耗损肾中精气，导致肾的阴阳失调，故中医认为久病脏腑受损，穷必及肾。

The term means that long-standing disease will eventually affect the kidney. From the perspective of traditional Chinese medicine (TCM), the kidney is the prenatal foundation. It stores innate essence and acquired essence. Its essential qi is the foundation of human life activities; its essence is the material basis for both kidney yin and kidney yang. Under normal physiological conditions, the kidney receives and stores the essential qi from the five *zang*-organs and six *fu*-organs. The remaining essential qi of the other *zang-fu* organs will be transmitted to and stored in the kidney except the consumed part in their own physical activities. Thus, the kidney is the storehouse of essential qi. When other *zang-fu* organs are impaired, leading to disharmony between yin and yang, the kidney will be eventually affected. For one thing, no essential qi will be transmitted to and stored in the kidney; for another, the kidney is expected to transmit its essential qi to other *zang-fu* organs to maintain a minimum level of functional activities. Prolonged morbidity may exhaust the essential qi of the kidney, causing the disharmony between kidney yin and kidney yang. Hence, TCM believes that prolonged morbidity affects *zang-fu* organs and, as a result, affects the kidney.

【曾经译法】无

【现行译法】无

【推荐译法】Prolonged morbidity affects the kidney.

【翻译说明】"穷必及肾"的意思是久病必然影响到肾。"穷"意为发展到最后，表示疾病病程长，可译为 prolonged morbidity；"及"意为累及、影响，可译为 affect。

引例 Citations:

◎ 虚邪之至，害必归阴，五脏之伤，穷必及肾。（《景岳全书·杂证谟》）

（病邪侵犯人体，必然会损伤阴精；五脏受到损伤，发展到最后必然影响到肾。）

When deficient pathogen invades the human body, yin will be impaired. When the five *zang*-organs are impaired, the kidney will be eventually affected. (*Complete Works of Jingyue*)

◎ 盖五志生火，动必关心，脏阴既伤，穷必及肾也。（《金匮要略心典》卷下）

（大概五志过极化生火热，火动必然影响到心，五脏之阴既然受伤，发展到最后必然影响到肾。）

Probably, when the excess of five emotions transforms into fire, its flaming will eventually affect the heart. When yin aspects of the five *zang*-organs are impaired, prolonged morbidity will eventually affect the kidney. (*Understanding of "Essential Prescriptions of the Golden Cabinet"*) bìngrùgāohuāng

# 病入膏肓

The Disease Has Attacked the Vitals.

古人以膏为心尖脂肪，肓为心脏与隔膜之间，膏肓之间是药力不到之处。病入膏肓，指疾病已经进入膏肓，形容病情极为严重，无法医治；也指事态极为严重，无法挽救。病入膏肓语出《左传·成公十年》，言晋景公病重，向秦国邀请良医来治病。秦桓公派医缓前来给晋景公治病。医缓尚未到达的时候，晋景公梦见自己的病变成了两个小孩儿，一个小孩儿说："医缓是个好医生，惧怕他伤害我们，我们往哪里逃跑呢？"另一个说："我们待在肓的上边，膏的下边，医缓能把我们怎么样？"医缓来到，看了病说："病不能治了。病在肓之上，膏之下，灸不能用，针达不到，药力又不能至，不能治了"。

The term means that the disease has invaded the fat of cardiac apex and the space between the heart and the diaphragm. It is believed by the ancient Chinese that no medicine could heal the disease located in the fat of cardiac apex and the space between the heart and the diaphragm, meaning that the illness is critical, or beyond cure. It also means that the problem is too serious to be solved. According to *Zuo's Commentary of the Spring and Autumn Annals*, the Duke Jing of the State of Jin developed a serious illness and asked the State of Qin to send a good doctor. Yi Huan was therefore requested by the Duke Huan of Qin to treat the disease. Before the arrival of Yi Huan, the Duke Jing of Jin dreamed that his illness had changed into two children. One of them said: "Yi Huan is a good doctor. What if he hurts us? Where can we escape?" The other said: "We can hide in the space between the heart and the diaphragm and below the cardiac apex. What can Yi Huan do about us?" When Yi Huan arrived, he examined the patient and said: "The disease is beyond cure. It is located in the space between the heart and the diaphragm and below the cardiac apex. Neither moxibustion, needling, nor medication can work. It is incurable."

【曾经译法】 the disease has attacked the vitals; being critically ill; disease beyond cure; disease reaching to (note: "to" should be deleted) the deepest heart, hopeless situation

【现行译法】 critical condition of disease; disease which has attacked vitals; being critically ill; disease involving Gao and Huang

【推荐译法】 The disease has attacked the vitals.

【翻译说明】 "膏"为心尖脂肪,"肓"为心脏与隔膜之间,"膏肓"指病位深隐,"病入膏肓"指疾病发展到了无法医治的地步,可译为 The disease has attacked the vitals,"vitals"表示"重要器官,命脉,要害"。根据上下文,也可采取意译。

引例 Citations:

◎ 脉但浮,时无里证表邪,犹合用麻黄,不尿,腹满犹加哕,关格之病入膏肓。(《普济方》卷一百二十五)

（脉只见浮象,没有里证和表邪,还合用麻黄,不排尿,腹满而且干呕,此乃关格病入膏肓。）

The patient has a floating pulse, yet without an interior pattern or exterior pathogens. Ephedra is used in combination. The patient has anuria, abdominal fullness, and retching. This is *Guan Ge* disorder (characterized by urinary block and vomiting) attacking the vitals. (*Formulas for Universal Relief*)

◎ 然患者亦当早治,勿待病入膏肓,虽有神丹亦无济也。(《重楼玉钥》卷上)

（但患者也应该早治,不要等到病入膏肓,否则即使有神丹也无济于事。）

However, treatment should be sought as early as possible. Do not wait until critical condition develops, when even magic pills cannot save lives. (*Jade Key to the Secluded Chamber*) guàibìng duō tán

# 怪病多痰

Rare or Difficult Diseases Are Most Likely Caused by Phlegm.

　　中医诊治奇难杂病的思路之一，言一些罕见的疑难病症多为痰所致。痰是人体水液代谢障碍所形成的病理产物，其形成之后，又可导致新的疾病发生，故痰既属于病理产物，又是致病因素。痰属阴邪，其性黏滞，可以阻碍气机，阻滞血行，由痰生瘀；痰致病部位十分广泛，内至脏腑，外至筋骨皮肉，无处不到，可影响多个脏腑组织；痰易蒙蔽清窍，扰乱神明，出现一系列神志失常的病症；痰邪致病病势缠绵，病程较长，难于速愈。正由于痰致病的广泛性、复杂性、顽固性，故中医有"百病皆由痰作祟""怪病多从痰着手"等说法。

The term reflects one of the ways of thinking in the diagnosis and treatment of rare or difficult diseases with traditional Chinese medicine (TCM). It means that some rare or difficult diseases are likely caused by phlegm. Phlegm is a pathological product of disrupted metabolism of the body fluids. Its formation may cause emerging diseases and it is a pathogenic factor as well. Phlegm is ascribed to yin pathogen. Sticky in nature, it may block the circulation of qi and blood and result in blood stasis. Phlegm may cause diseases in a variety of body parts, from the inner *zang-fu* organs to tendons, bones, skins, as well as muscles and flesh. It may occur anywhere, affecting multiple tissues and *zang-fu* organs. Phlegm is likely to obstruct orifices, disturb the mind, and cause a series of mental disorders. Phlegm-related diseases tend to linger for a long time, and are difficult to cure. Because of the extensiveness, complexity, and intractability of those disorders, TCM believes that "all diseases are caused by phlegm" and "the factor of phlegm should first be considered in treating rare or difficult diseases."

【曾经译法】无

【现行译法】rare disease often caused by phlegm

【推荐译法】 Rare or difficult diseases are most likely caused by phlegm.

【翻译说明】 术语中的"多"可理解为"多半"，表示有较大可能性，可译为 most likely。"怪病"表示"罕见的疑难病症"，可译为 rare or difficult diseases。推荐译法相比于现行译法表述更为严谨。

引例 Citations:

◎ 暴病之谓火，怪病之谓痰。(《仁斋直指附遗方论》卷一)

    (忽然发生的疾病多属于火，罕见的疑难病症多属于痰。)

Sudden disease emergence is most likely caused by fire; rare or difficult diseases are most likely caused by phlegm. (*Discussion on Supplements to "Renzhai's Direct Guidance on Formulas"*)

◎ 天下怪病多生于痰，而痰病多成于湿痰。(《辨证录》卷二)

    (所有的怪病多因痰而发，痰病大多因湿痰而形成。)

Rare or difficult diseases are most likely caused by phlegm. Phlegm diseases are most likely caused by dampness phlegm. (*Records on Syndrome Differentiation*) shòurén duō huǒ

# 瘦人多火

Thin People Tend to Have Internal Fire.

瘦人多火，指形体消瘦的人，由于精血、津液等物质不足，阴液亏少，阴不制阳，脏腑功能偏亢而阳有余，故其人火旺。形瘦阴亏之人，易感温热阳邪，而愈使其脏腑功能亢进，发病后易出现火热之证。故临床上对体质偏瘦的患者，诊治时要考虑素体有火的因素，治疗时多以滋阴清热为法，用药多偏寒凉，或清热泻火，或滋阴降火。瘦人多火，切忌辛热温燥之品，以防更伤其阴，助阳化火。同时亦忌辛辣之物，因其皆可耗阴，助热化火。

The term means that people of slight build are likely to have internal fire due to insufficiency of blood and body fluids resulting in yin deficiency, causing yang excess and hyperactivity of *zang-fu* organs as a result of yin being unable to restrain yang. Thin people with yin deficiency are apt to be affected by warm-heat yang pathogen. They tend to have hyperactivity of *zang-fu* organs and fire-heat patterns after a pathogen attack. When diagnosing and treating thin people, fire aspect should be considered. The method of nourishing yin and clearing heat is often used. Medicines with cold or cool property are often prescribed, either to clear heat to purge fire or to nourish yin to reduce fire. Since thin people tend to have internal fire, they should avoid pungency, hotness, warmness, and dryness to prevent yang from transforming into fire due to further impairment of yin. They should also avoid pungent and spicy foods because these foods may consume yin and facilitate heat to transform into fire.

【曾经译法】无

【现行译法】thin people tend to have internal heat; thin persons are subject to vigorous fire

【推荐译法】Thin people tend to have internal fire.

【翻译说明】术语中的"多"可理解为"多半"，表示有较大可能性。英文短语 tend to do sth. 表示有很大可能性发生，契合术语含义。

引例 Citations:

◎ 不可拘肥人多痰，瘦人多火，而以燥湿泻火之药轻治之也。（《妇人良方大全》卷一）

（不可拘泥于肥人多痰，瘦人多火的观点，而用燥湿泻火的药物，用量较小地治疗。）

Don't be limited by the thoughts that obese people tend to have phlegm and that thin people tend to have internal fire. Rather, use medicines that can dry dampness and purge fire at a lower dose to treat. (*The Complete Compendium of Fine Formulas for Women*)

◎ 况瘦人多火，又加泄精，则水益少而火益炽。（《辨证录》卷十一）

（况且瘦人多火，又加之精液外泄，就会使水更少而火更旺。）

Additionally, thin people tend to have internal fire. When their kidney essence leaks, the kidney water becomes even less and fire is further stoked. (*Records on Syndrome Differentiation*) féirén duō tán

# 肥人多痰

Obese People Tend to Have Phlegm.

肥人多痰，是指形体肥胖的人，体内多痰湿内盛，形成痰湿体质。痰湿是由于津液输布、排泄障碍，水湿蓄积于体内而形成的病理产物。痰湿的形成，从脏腑角度来说，与脾肾阳气不足，蒸腾气化失司关系密切。肥胖体质者，常伴有不同程度的阳气虚弱，阳气温运阴津不及，水湿停聚不化而为痰饮；且肥胖阳虚之人，对寒湿阴邪又较易感，故临床上肥人多见痰饮、水肿等水湿之邪为患。诊治时须考虑其气虚湿邪痰饮的因素，治疗多用温阳散寒、健脾利湿等法，用药多以温燥、芳化、渗湿为主。切忌用寒凉之药损伤阳气，或肥甘厚腻之品损伤脾胃，助湿生痰。

The term means that obese persons are apt to have phlegm-dampness constitution due to excess phlegm dampness in the body. Phlegm is a pathological product of water-dampness retention as a result of disrupted distribution and excretion of body fluids. From the perspective of *zang-fu* organs, it is closely associated with insufficiency of spleen-kidney yang and the latter's failure in vaporizing and transforming qi. Obese people often have varying degrees of yang deficiency so that their yang qi is not sufficient to warm and transport yin fluids, causing water-dampness retention, and then phlegm-dampness accumulation. Obese persons with yang deficiency are apt to be affected by yin pathogens of cold and dampness. In clinical practice, invasion of water dampness, e.g., phlegm and edema, is commonly found in obese patients. Factors such as qi deficiency, dampness, and phlegm should be considered in disease diagnosis and treatment. Warming yang to dissipate cold and strengthening the spleen to remove dampness are often used. Medicines are primarily prescribed to warm dryness, resolve dampness with warm, dry and aromatic herbs. Medicines with cold or cool property should be avoided in case they impair yang qi. Greasy and sweet food should be avoided as they may impair the spleen-stomach function and contribute to the transformation of dampness into phlegm.

【曾经译法】 patient with obesity tend to have copious phlegm

【现行译法】 obese people tending to have copious phlegm; patient with obesity tend to have copious phlegm

【推荐译法】 Obese people tend to have phlegm.

【翻译说明】 "肥人"指形体肥胖的人，建议译为 obese people，而不是 patient with obesity（肥胖症患者）。"多痰"可理解为体内多痰湿内盛。为照顾类似术语结构翻译的一致性，建议将"肥人多痰"译为 Obese people tend to have phlegm。


引例 Citations:


◎ 肥人多痰，年高必用人捶而痛快者，属痰属虚，除湿化痰，兼补脾肾。（《医学六要·治法汇》）

（肥胖的人多痰病，年龄大须让人捶背而感觉痛快者，属于痰证虚证，治疗宜除湿化痰，兼补益脾肾。）

Obese people tend to have phlegm. Senior patients will feel relieved after being thumped on the back, an indication of phlegm patterns and deficiency patterns. The treatment should be eliminating dampness and resolving phlegm as well as tonifying the spleen and the kidney simultaneously. (*Six Essentials of Medicine*)

◎ 肥人多痰乃气虚也，虚则气不能运行，故痰生之。（《石室秘录》卷三）

（肥胖的人多痰是由于气虚所致，气虚不能正常运行，因此产生痰。）

It is due to qi deficiency that obese people tend to have phlegm. Deficiency results in disrupted flow of qi, thus causing phlegm. (*Secret Records in a Stone Room*)

bāgāng

# 八纲

Eight Principles

八纲，即表、里、寒、热、虚、实、阴、阳八个辨证的纲领。八纲是从临床错综复杂的病证中抽象出来的、带有普遍规律的证候，是中医辨证的纲领，较为突出地反映了中医学的辩证法思想。其中，疾病病位的浅深可分为表证和里证，疾病的性质可区分为寒证和热证，邪正的盛衰可概括为实证和虚证，疾病的类别可归属于阳证和阴证两大类。八纲辨证就是将疾病错综复杂的临床表现，归纳为表与里、寒与热、虚与实、阴与阳四对纲领性证候，用于指导临床治疗。其中阴阳又是总纲，它可以概括其他六纲，即里、虚、寒证属阴证；表、实、热证属阳证。因此，八纲辨证是分析疾病共性的辨证方法，在临床诊断过程中，具有执简驭繁、提纲挈领的作用。

The eight principles are used to guide identification of patterns including interior, exterior, cold, heat, deficiency, excess, yin, and yang. Abstracted from complex clinical manifestations, these principles are universal and regarded as the guidelines for pattern differentiation. They present a good example of dialectic thinking in traditional Chinese medicine. Using these parameters, one could determine the disease location (exterior or interior), nature (heat or cold), the situation of predominance of pathogenic factors (excess) or lack of healthy qi (deficiency), and the overall type of diseases (yang or yin). The eight principles classify various clinical conditions into four pairs of patterns, i.e., interior and exterior, cold and heat, deficiency and excess, and yin and yang, to guide clinical treatment. Yin and yang are the leading principles. They sum up the remaining ones: interior, deficiency, and cold disorders are yin; exterior, excess, and heat disorders are yang. Therefore, the common characteristics of diseases can be analyzed in terms of the eight principles that concentrate on the essential points. They are brief and explicit, playing a fundamental role in clinical diagnosis.

【曾经译法】 eight principles

【现行译法】 (the) eight principles; the eight guiding principles; eight diagnostic principles

【推荐译法】 eight principles

【翻译说明】 "八纲"的译法比较一致，考虑术语简洁性原则，建议译为 eight principles。

引例 Citations:

◎ 仲景治伤寒，着三百九十七法，一百一十三方……然究其大要，无出乎表、里、虚、实、阴、阳、寒、热八者而已。(《医林绳墨》)

（张仲景治疗伤寒病用 397 法，113 个方剂……但总括其大要，无外乎表、里、虚、实、阴、阳、寒、热八个方面。）

A total of 397 methods including 113 formulas were used by Zhang Zhongjing to treat cold damage… Nevertheless, they boil down to eight parameters: interior, exterior, deficiency, excess, yin, yang, cold, and heat. (*Standardized Medical Treatments*)

◎ 所谓八纲者，阴阳、表里、寒热、虚实是也。古昔医工，观察各种疾病之征候，就其性能之不同，归纳于八种纲要，执简驭繁，以应无穷之变。(《伤寒质难》)

（所谓八纲，就是阴阳、表里、寒热、虚实。古代医生观察各种疾病之证候，根据其性态的不同，归纳为八种纲要，执简驭繁，以应无穷变化。）

The eight principles refer to yin, yang, interior, exterior, cold, heat, deficiency, and excess. Ancient physicians categorized various disorders in terms of eight parameters according to their nature. The eight principles focus on the essential points, catering to infinite variety. (*Challenges to Cold Damage*) fēngzhèng

# 风证

Wind Pattern/Syndrome

风证，指风邪侵袭人体肌表、经络，卫外功能失常所引起的证候。临床表现为恶风，微发热，汗出，头痛，鼻塞，流清涕，喷嚏，咽喉痒痛，干咳，舌苔薄白，脉浮缓；或突起风团，皮肤瘙痒，瘾疹；或突发肌肤麻木，口眼歪斜；或肌肉强直、痉挛，抽搐；或肢体关节游走作痛；或新起面睑、肢体浮肿等。辨证要点为恶风，微热，汗出，脉浮缓；或突起风团，瘙痒，麻木，肢体关节游走疼痛，面睑浮肿等。

The term refers to the pattern or syndrome caused by defense qi failing to protect the human body due to wind invading the body surface, meridians, and collaterals. Clinical manifestations include an aversion to wind, slight fever, sweating, headache, nasal obstruction, a runny nose, sneezing, painful and itching throat, dry cough, a thin white tongue coating, and a floating, slowdown pulse. It may also manifest the following groups of symptoms: a sudden onset of wheals, skin itching or rashes; sudden numbness of the skin, facial paralysis; muscle stiffness, spasms, and convulsions; migratory joint pains; newly-formed edema in the face, eyelids, and limbs. Key points of differentiation are an aversion to wind, slight fever, sweating, and a floating, slow-down pulse; or a sudden onset of wheals, local itching, numbness, migratory joint pains, and facial and eyelid edemas.

【曾经译法】 wind syndrome

【现行译法】 wind syndrome; wind syndrome/pattern; wind pattern

【推荐译法】 wind pattern/syndrome

【翻译说明】"证"指证候，是疾病所处一定阶段本质的反映，或对一定阶段的某种类型的病因、病性、病位等的概括，包含患者的临床表现、对病机的判断以及诊断结论，常译为 pattern，有时也译为 syndrome。"风证"的译法比较一致，常译为 wind pattern/syndrome。

引例 Citations:

◎ 附香散治中风偏痹，经络不通，手足缓弱，臂膝酸疼，凡风证始作，脉息不洪数者，先宜服此药。(《杨氏家藏方》卷一)

（附香散治疗中风肢体一侧痹阻，经络不通，手足缓弱，上下肢酸疼，凡风证开始发作，脉无洪数之象，先宜服用此药。）

*Fu Xiang* Powder (Powder of Aconite and Aucklandia Root) is used to remove blockage on one side of the body due to wind stroke, obstruction of meridians and collaterals, slowness and weakness of hands and feet, as well as soreness and pain of the extremities. It is appropriate to take this medicine first at the onset of wind pattern when the pulse is not surging or rapid. (*Reserved Formulas of Yang's Family*)

◎ 若湿气胜，风证不退，眩运麻木不已，除风湿羌活汤主之。(《脾胃论》卷中)

（假若湿气偏胜，风证不退，眩晕、麻木不除，治疗用除风湿羌活汤。）

*Chu Fengshi Qianghuo* Decoction (Notopterygium Decoction for Expelling Wind Dampness) is used when dampness is predominant, wind pattern does not subside, and symptoms of vertigo and numbness remain. (*Treatise on the Spleen and Stomach*)

# 寒证

Cold Pattern/Syndrome

寒证，指寒邪侵袭机体，阳气被遏，或阳虚阴盛引起的证候。临床表现为恶寒重，或伴发热，无汗，头身疼痛，鼻塞，流清涕，脉浮紧；或见咳嗽，哮喘，咯稀白痰；或为脘腹疼痛，肠鸣腹泻，呕吐；或为四肢厥冷，局部拘急冷痛等。口不渴或渴喜热饮，小便清长，面色苍白，舌苔白，脉弦紧或沉迟。辨证要点为恶寒肢冷，无汗，局部冷痛，苔白，脉紧或沉迟等。

The term refers to the pattern or syndrome caused by yang qi being suppressed or the situation of yang deficiency and yin excess due to invasion of cold on the body surface. Clinical manifestations include severe aversion to cold with or without fever, absence of sweating, head and body ache, nasal obstruction, a runny nose, and a floating, tight pulse. It may also manifest the following groups of symptoms: cough, asthma, and thin white sputum; epigastric pain, intestinal rumblings, diarrhea, and vomiting; cold limbs, local cramps, and cold pain; no desire to drink or preference for hot drinks, clear and profuse urine, pale complexion, a white tongue coating, and a wiry, tight pulse or a deep, slow pulse. Key points of differentiation are aversion to cold, cold limbs, no sweating, local cold pain, a white tongue coating, and a tight pulse or a deep, slow pulse.

【曾经译法】 cold-syndrome; cold syndrome; cold pattern

【现行译法】 cold syndrome/syndrome of cold type; cold syndrome/pattern; cold pattern

【推荐译法】 cold pattern/syndrome

【翻译说明】 "证"指证候，是疾病所处一定阶段本质的反映，或对一定阶段的某种类型的病因、病性、病位等的概括，包含患者的临床表现、对病机的判断以及诊断结论，常译为 pattern，有时也会译为 syndrome。"寒证"的译法比较一致，常译为 cold pattern/syndrome。

引例 Citations:

◎ 寒则腹痛而啼，面青白，口有冷气，腹亦冷，曲腰而啼，此寒证也。（《三因极一病证方论》卷十八）

（寒性则腹痛啼哭，面色青白，口中出冷气，腹部也冷，弯腰啼哭，这是寒证。）

The cold nature of a disease is characterized by cries due to abdominal pain, bluish and pale complexion, cold breath coming out of the mouth, cold abdomen, and stooping to cry. These indicate a cold pattern. (*Discussion of Pathology Based on Triple Etiology Doctrine*)

◎ 外感宜泻，而内伤宜补，寒证可温，而热证可清。（《仁斋直指附遗方论》卷一）

（外感病证宜用泻法，内伤病证宜用补法，寒证可以温，热证可以清。）

Externally contracted disorders should be treated by purging, whereas endogenous injury should be treated by tonifying. Cold patterns can be treated by warming, whereas heat patterns can be treated by clearing. (*Discussion on Supplements to "Renzhai's Direct Guidance on Formulas"*)

# 暑证

Summer-heat Pattern/Syndrome

暑证，指感受暑热之邪所引起的证候。临床表现为发热恶热，心烦汗出，口渴喜饮，气短神疲，肢体困倦，小便短黄，舌红，苔白或黄，脉虚数；或发热，胸闷脘痞，腹痛，呕恶，无汗，苔黄腻，脉濡数；或发热，猝然昏倒，汗出不止，气急；甚至昏迷、抽搐，舌绛干燥，脉细数等。辨证要点为有夏季感受暑热之邪的病史，以发热、汗出、口渴、疲乏、尿黄等为主要表现。

The term refers to the pattern or syndrome caused by invasion of summer heat. Clinical manifestations include fever yet with an aversion to heat, vexation, sweating, thirst and preference for drinks, shortness of breath, fatigue, physical drowsiness, scanty and yellow urine, a red tongue, a white or yellow tongue coating, and a deficient, rapid pulse. It may also manifest the following groups of symptoms: fever, chest tightness, stomach stuffiness, abdominal pain, nausea, absence of sweating, a yellow, greasy tongue coating, and a soft, rapid pulse; fever, sudden syncope, persistent sweating, and rapid breathing; or even coma, convulsions, a crimson and dry tongue, and a thready, rapid pulse. The key point of differentiation is a history of being invaded by summer heat characterized by fever, sweating, thirst, fatigue, and yellow urine.

【曾经译法】 heat stroke (暑); summerheat (暑)

【现行译法】 summer-heat syndrome; summer-heat syndrome/pattern; syndrome of summerheat; summer heat pattern; summerheat syndrome; summerheat pattern/syndrome; summer syndrome; syndrome/pattern of summer-heat

【推荐译法】 summer-heat pattern/syndrome

【翻译说明】 "证" 指证候，是疾病所处一定阶段本质的反映，或对一定阶段的某种类型的病因、病性、病位等的概括，包含患者的临床表现、对病机的判断以及诊断结论，常译为 pattern，有时也译为 syndrome。"暑证"可译为 summer-heat pattern/syndrome。

引例 Citations:

◎ 六和汤，治暑证身热，呕不甚渴。(《仁斋直指附遗方论》卷三)

（六和汤，治疗暑证身体发热，呕吐，口不太渴。）

*Liu He* Decoction (Mixed Decoction of Six Ingredients) is used to treat summer-heat disorders such as increased body temperature, vomiting, and mild thirst. (*Discussion on Supplements to "Renzhai's Direct Guidance on Formulas"*)

◎ 暑证用黄连香薷饮，挟痰加半夏南星，如虚加参芪。(《丹溪心法附余》卷二)

（治疗暑证用黄连香薷饮，挟痰者加半夏、天南星，若气虚加人参、黄芪。）

*Huanglian Xiangru* Drink (Coptis and Elshotzia Drink) is used to treat summer-heat disorders. *Banxia* (*Rhizoma Pinelliae*, Pinellia Tuber) and *tiannanxing* (*Rhizoma Arisaematis*, Jack-in-the-Pulpit Tuber) are added when the patient has phlegm; *renshen* (*Radix Ginseng*, Ginseng) and *huangqi* (*Radix Astragali*, astragalus root) are added when the patient has qi deficiency. (*Appendices to Danxi's Experiential Therapy*) shīzhèng

# 湿证

Dampness Pattern/Syndrome

湿证，指感受湿邪，阻遏人体气机与清阳所引起的证候。临床表现为头重如裹，肢体困重，倦怠嗜睡，面色晦垢，舌苔滑腻，脉濡缓或细。或伴恶寒发热，或肢体关节、肌肉酸痛，或为局部渗漏湿液，或皮肤湿疹、瘙痒；胸闷脘痞，口腻不渴，纳呆恶心，腹胀腹痛，大便稀溏，小便混浊；妇女可见带下量多。辨证要点为身体困重、酸楚，痞闷，腻浊，脉濡缓等。

The term refers to the pattern or syndrome caused by blockage of qi activity and clear yang due to invasion of dampness. Clinical manifestations include head heaviness as if being wrapped up, limb heaviness, lethargy, hypersomnia, dark and lusterless complexion, a slippery, greasing tongue coating, and a soft, slowdown pulse or a thready pulse. It may also manifest the following groups of symptoms: an aversion to cold, fever; limb joint and muscle pains, soreness; local leakage of moisture; skin eczema and itching; chest tightness, stomach stuffiness, greasiness in the mouth with no desire to drink, poor appetite, nausea, abdominal distention, abdominal pain, loose stools, and turbid urine. Women may have profuse leukorrhea. Key points of differentiation are heaviness in the body, soreness, stuffiness, tightness, greasy and turbid sensations, and a soft, slowdown pulse.

【曾经译法】无

【现行译法】damp syndrome; damp(ness) syndrome/pattern; dampness pattern

【推荐译法】dampness pattern/syndrome

【翻译说明】"证"指证候，是疾病所处一定阶段本质的反映，或对一定阶段的某种类型的病因、病性、病位等的概括，包含患者的临床表现、对病机的判断以及诊断结论，常译为pattern，有时也译为 syndrome。"湿"采用名词形式，译为 dampness。
"湿证"常译为 dampness pattern/syndrome。

引例 Citations:

◎ 五苓散治湿证小便不利，经云治湿之法不利小便，非其治也。（《仁斋直指方》卷三）

（五苓散治疗湿证小便不利，《素问病机气宜保命集》言治湿之法不通利小便，不是治湿的方法。）

*Wu Ling* Powder (Five-ingredient Powder with Poria) is used to treat inhibited urination due to dampness patterns. According to "Collection of Writings on the Mechanism of Disease, Suitability of Qi, and the Safeguarding of Life" in *Plain Conversation*, the method of removing dampness has to involve promoting urination. (*Renzhai's Direct Guidance on Formulas*)

◎ 湿证虽多，而辨治之法，其要惟二：则一曰湿热，一曰寒湿而尽之矣。（《景岳全书·杂证谟》）

（湿证临床虽多，但辨治的方法，其要点只有两个：一是湿热，一是寒湿，即可全部概括。）

Although dampness patterns encompass a variety of disorders, there are basically two essential points for differentiation: dampness heat and cold dampness. All signs and symptoms can be classified into these two aspects. (*Complete Works of Jingyue*) zàozhèng

# 燥证

Dryness Pattern/Syndrome

燥证，指外感燥邪，耗伤津液引起的证候。临床表现为口唇、鼻腔、咽喉干燥，皮肤干燥甚至皲裂、脱屑，口渴欲饮，舌苔干燥，大便干燥，小便短黄，或见干咳少痰，痰黏难咯等。属于温燥者常兼见发热微恶风寒，有汗，咽喉疼痛，舌边尖红，脉浮数；属于凉燥者常兼有恶寒发热，无汗，头痛，脉浮紧。辨证要点为时值秋季或处于气候干燥的环境，具有干燥不润的证候特点。

The term refers to the pattern or syndrome caused by fluid consumption due to exogenous dryness. Clinical manifestations include dryness of the mouth, lips, nose, and throat, dry, rough, and even chapped skin with scaling, thirst with a desire to drink, a dry tongue coating, dry stools, scanty yellow urine, or dry cough with a small amount of sticky sputum difficult to expectorate. Warm-dryness cases may also manifest fever, mild aversion to wind and cold, sweating, sore throat, red tongue tip and sides, and a floating, rapid pulse. Cool-dryness cases may manifest an aversion to cold, fever, absence of sweating, headache, and a floating, tight pulse. Key points of differentiation are dryness and lack of moisture due to the autumn season or a dry climate.

【曾经译法】dryness syndrome

【现行译法】dryness syndrome; dryness pattern

【推荐译法】dryness pattern/syndrome

【翻译说明】"证"指证候，是疾病所处一定阶段本质的反映，或对一定阶段的某种类型的病因、病性、病位等的概括，包含患者的临床表现、对病机的判断以及诊断结论，常译为 pattern，有时也译为 syndrome。"燥证"常译为 dryness pattern/syndrome。

引例 Citations:

◎ 岁金太过，至秋深燥金用事，久晴不雨，得燥证，皮肤拆裂，手足枯燥，搔之屑起。(《医学正传》卷二)

（金运太过，到深秋燥气主事，久晴不下雨，患燥证，见皮肤开裂，手足枯燥，搔抓则起皮屑。）

Metal (lung) phase is excessive. When late autumn arrives, dryness takes dominance and sunny days persist for a long time without rainfall. Dryness patterns occur, usually manifested as chapped skin, dry hands and feet, and scaling upon scratching. (*Orthodoxy of Medicine*)

◎ 凡治杂病，有兼带燥证者，误用燥药，转成其燥，因致危困者，医之罪也。(《医门法律》卷三)

（凡治疗杂病，对兼有燥证的患者，若误用燥性的药物，则使燥证加重，由此导致病情危重，这是医生的过错。）

The dryness pattern will be aggravated and a critical condition will occur if the physician misuses medicines with dry property to treat patients with miscellaneous diseases accompanied by dryness disorders. In such cases, the physician is at fault. (*Precepts for Physicians*) huǒzhèng

# 火证

Fire Pattern/Syndrome

火证，指外感火热之邪，或饮食不当、情志过极或阴虚阳亢，导致阳热内盛引起的证候。临床表现为发热恶热，烦躁，口渴喜饮，汗多，大便秘结，小便短黄，面色赤，舌红或绛，苔黄而干或灰黑干燥，脉洪滑数。甚则神昏、谵语，惊厥抽搐，吐血，衄血，痈肿疮疡。火热证有表里虚实之分。表热多有兼夹他邪而出现风热、暑热、燥热等证。里热属实证，有肺热炽盛、心火亢盛、胃热炽盛、热扰胸膈、肠热腑实、肝火上炎、肝火犯肺、热入营血证等。辨证要点为新病突起，病势较剧，以发热、口渴、便秘、尿黄、出血、舌红苔黄、脉数为主要表现。

The term refers to the pattern or syndrome caused by excess yang heat in the body due to invasion of fire heat, improper diet, extreme emotions, or the disorder of yin deficiency and yang hyperactivity. Clinical manifestations include fever, an aversion to heat, vexation, thirst and preference for drinks, profuse sweating, constipation, scanty yellow urine, red complexion, a red or crimson tongue with a yellow or a grayish-black dry coating, and a surging, slippery, rapid pulse. In severe cases, patients will manifest unconsciousness, delirium, convulsions, blood vomiting, nosebleeds, carbuncles, and sores. Fire-heat pattern is classified into the types of exterior, interior, deficiency, and excess. Exterior heat, usually accompanied by other pathogenic factors, is characterized by wind heat, summer heat, and dryness heat. Interior heat is an excess pattern, characterized by excessive lung heat, hyperactive heart fire, excessive stomach heat, heat disturbing chest and diaphragm, intestinal heat and excess *fu*-organs, flaring liver fire, liver fire invading the lung, and heat entering the nutrient and blood aspects. Key points of differentiation are a sudden onset of emerging acute diseases, characterized by fever, thirst, constipation, yellow urine, bleeding, a red tongue with a yellow coating, and a rapid pulse.

【曾经译法】 fire syndrome

【现行译法】 fire syndrome; fire pattern

【推荐译法】 fire pattern/syndrome

【翻译说明】 "证"指证候，是疾病所处一定阶段本质的反映，或对一定阶段的某种类型的病因、病性、病位等的概括，包含患者的临床表现、对病机的判断以及诊断结论，常译为 pattern，有时也译为 syndrome。"火证"常译为 fire pattern/syndrome。


引例 Citations:


◎ 水火人身之阴阳也，阳常有余，故火证恒多。(《济阳纲目》卷二十五)

　　(水火乃人身之阴阳，阳常有余，因此火证经常较多。)

Fire and water are yang and yin in the human body. Yang is usually in excess, hence there are more fire patterns. (*Guide to Saving Yang*)

◎ 火证有实火者焉，心火燔灼，胃火助之，而元气未损，真精未亏。(《医学入门衡要》卷二)

　　(火证有属于实火者，心火燔灼，胃火辅助，但元气尚未损伤，精气尚未亏虚。)

Fire patterns can be excess, with symptoms of flaring heart fire and aiding stomach fire, but the original qi is not impaired and the essential qi is not deficient yet. (*An Introduction to Medicine: Selected Essentials*) màizhèng-hécān

# 脉证合参

Analysis of Both Pulse Conditions and Symptoms

脉证合参，指辨证过程中把脉象与患者的异常感觉或某些病态改变互相参照以推断病情的方法。由于古代证、症不分，均用"证"字，故现代又称"脉症合参"。脉象本来也是一种体征，只是一种比较独特的诊法，具有比较特殊的意义，故中医学将脉象与其他体征、症状等同视之，强调脉与体征、症状在诊断中具有同等重要的地位。由于同一种脉象可见于多种不同病证，而同一病证也可出现多种不同的脉象，因此，脉与证密切相关，不可离开证去论脉，也不可离开脉去论证，只有脉证合参，知常达变，方可辨证无误。一般来说，脉证属性一致为顺，相反为逆。

The terms refers to the method of diagnosing medical conditions by cross-referencing the pulse conditions with the patient's unwell feelings or certain pathological changes in the process of pattern identification. In ancient times, no distinction was made between *zheng* (证, pattern or syndrome) and *zheng* (症, symptom). Hence, the latter is used as an alternative to the former in modern times. Pulse condition is a sign; pulse-feeling is a unique diagnostic method with added value. Traditional Chinese medicine regards pulse conditions as important as other signs and symptoms, emphasizing in diagnosis the equal value of pulse conditions, signs, and symptoms. The same pulse can be found in many different patterns, and the same pattern can manifest a variety of pulse conditions; therefore, pulse conditions and patterns are closely related. Both should be considered in diagnosis. Only when pulse conditions and patterns are combined for analysis can one discern changes by measuring against the normal and avoid mistakes in pattern identification. Generally, when the nature of a pulse is consistent with that of signs and symptoms, it is conformity. Otherwise, it is adversity.

【曾经译法】 comprehensive analysis to (note: "to" should be revised as "of") the patient's pulse condition and symptoms; pulse combined with symptoms and signs; comprehensive analysis of pulse condition and other manifestations; making a diagnosis in the light of both pulse condition and symptoms observed; diagnosis by both pulse and symptoms; correlate pulse and symptoms; correlation of the pulse and symptoms; synthetical analysis of pulse and syndrome; synthesis of the pulse and symptoms

【现行译法】 considering pulse condition and symptoms in diagnosis of a disease; synthetical analysis of pulse and symptoms/diagnosis made in light of both pulse conditions and symptoms; consideration of both pulse and symptoms; Mutual combination of pulse and syndrome; pulse combined with symptoms and signs; comprehensive analysis of pulse and symptoms; synthetic analysis of pulse and symptoms; comprehensive analysis of the pulse quality and syndrome; comprehensive analysis of the pulse and symptoms; comprehensive analysis to (note: "to" should be revised as "of") both pulse manifestation and symptoms

【推荐译法】 analysis of both pulse conditions and symptoms

【翻译说明】 "脉"为脉象，2022 年发布的《世界卫生组织中医药术语国际标准》将此术语翻译为 pulse conditions。因此，建议将"脉证合参"译为 analysis of both pulse conditions and symptoms。


引例 Citations:


◎ 恙经半载，脉证合参，究属质亏烦劳，以致坎离不交。(《杏轩医案》卷三)

（疾病经过半年，脉证合参，最终诊断为体质亏虚而烦劳，以致心肾不交。）

Half a year later, after an analysis of both pulse conditions and symptoms, the disorder was eventually diagnosed as disharmony between the heart and the kidney as a result of weak constitution and overstrain. (*Cheng Xingxuan's Case Records*)

◎ 脉证合参，乃气结在上，津不运行，蒸变浊痰，由无形渐变有形。（《柳选四家医案·评选静香楼医案》）

（脉证合参，诊断为气阻滞在上，津液不能运行，热蒸变化为浊痰，由无形逐渐变为有形。）

An analysis of both pulse conditions and symptoms indicates that qi stagnates in the upper part of the body leading to disrupted flow of body fluids, and fluid retention (the intangible) transforms into turbid phlegm (the tangible) upon steaming. (*Case Records of Four Doctors Selected by Liu Baozhi*) nìliú-wǎnzhōu

# 逆流挽舟

Boat Against the Current for Relief

逆流挽舟，是指用疏散表邪的方药治疗外感夹湿痢疾的方法。清代喻嘉言始创此名，理论源于《黄帝内经》有关表里先后治法之论，以及张仲景、张从正等下痢论治的经验，为痢疾的治疗提供了新思路。本法适应于痢疾的两种情况：一是外感性下痢，其病机主要为邪气下陷，治疗机理为引邪出表；二是内伤性下痢，其病机主要为阳气下陷，治疗机理为升阳和解。临床见下痢脓血，里急后重，兼见恶寒发热、头痛、身痛、无汗、脉浮等，采用升散和扶正逐邪药物，使陷里之邪从表而解，代表方如人参败毒散、仓廪汤。

The term refers to the method of relieving dysentery due to exogenous dampness with medicines for dispelling exterior pathogens. Yu Jiayan of the Qing Dynasty first created this method. He drew it from the successive treatment of the exterior and the interior in *Huangdi's Inner Canon of Medicine*, and from the clinical experience of well-known physicians such as Zhang Zhongjing and Zhang Congzheng in treating dysentery. This therapeutic method provides a new insight into the treatment of dysentery. It is applicable to the following two conditions: dysentery caused by exogenous pathogens and that by internal dysfunction. The former is characterized by the sinking of pathogenic qi, and therefore its treatment aims to expel pathogens from the skin surface. The latter is characterized by the sinking of yang qi, and therefore its treatment aims to promote yang qi for harmonization. Clinical manifestations include dysentery with pus and blood, tenesmus, coupled with an aversion to cold, fever, headache, body aches, absence of sweating, and a floating pulse. Medicines for lifting, dissipating, and strengthening the body resistance are used to expel from the superficies the pathogenic factors that sink in the interior. Representative formulas include *Renshen Baidu* Powder (Ginseng Powder to Overcome Pathogenic Factors) and *Canglin* Decoction (Rice Granary Decoction).

【曾经译法】 boating up the river; save a boat in adverse current; boating up the stream; hauling the boat upstream; application of pungent-cool diaphoretics for dysentery

【现行译法】 boating-up-the-stream therapy (a treatment for dysentery at early stage by application of drugs for both expelling the superficial pathogenic factors and eliminating damp-heat); rowing upstream; Rowing up the stream; Propelling Boat against the Current; boating up the river; application of pungent-cool diaphoretics for dysentery; boating up the stream; boating up stream; tracking boat upstream (stopping diarrhea by diaphoresis); rowing upstream

【推荐译法】 boat against the current for relief

【翻译说明】 "逆流挽舟"是比喻说法，表示用疏散表邪的方药治疗外感夹湿痢疾。为体现中医取象比类的思维方法，同时又符合英语表达习惯，建议将之译为 boat against the current for relief。

引例 Citations:

◎ 故虽百日之远，仍用逆流挽舟之法，引其邪而出之于外。(《医学从众录》卷五)

（因此，虽然患病有百日之久，仍用逆流挽舟的治法，引导邪气从外而出。）

Therefore, the method of boating against the current for relief is still used to expel pathogenic qi from the superficies, though the disease has prolonged for a hundred days. (*Records of Following Others in Medicine*)

◎ 外邪内陷而为痢，必用逆流挽舟之法，引其邪而出于外，人参败毒散主之。(《血证论》卷四)

（外感邪气内陷而导致痢疾，必须用逆流挽舟的治法，引导邪气从外而出，方用人参败毒散。）

The method of boating against the current for relief must be used to expel pathogenic qi from the superficies in the treatment for dysentery due to the sinking of exogenous pathogens. *Renshen Baidu* Powder (Ginseng Powder to Overcome Pathogenic Factors) is used. (*Treatise on Blood Syndromes*) tíhú-jiēgài

# 提壶揭盖

Lift a Kettle and Remove Its Lid

提壶揭盖，原指盛满水的茶壶，要想使水顺利地倒出来，就必须在壶盖上凿个洞或把壶盖揭开。中医学家采用取象比类的方法，类推指开宣肺气而通利水道，以治疗癃闭、水肿等病症的方法。中医学认为肺位最高，为"华盖"，主宣发肃降、通调水道，为"水之上源"，对津液的输布、运行和排泄都具有推动作用。如果肺的宣发肃降功能失常，就会影响水液的代谢。肺失宣发，则影响水液外达皮肤，可见无汗、水肿等症；肺失肃降，则影响水液下输膀胱，可见小便不利和水肿等。治疗采用宣利肺气以通调水道的方法，代表方如越婢加术汤等。

The term literally means that a small hole should be made in the lid of a kettle or its lid should be removed when you pour out water from a full kettle through its spout. It is used analogically by traditional Chinese medicine (TCM) physicians to refer to the method of ventilating the lung to regulate water pathways in the treatment for disorders such as inhibited urination and edema. TCM believes that the lung, like a "florid canopy," locates at the highest part of the chest. It governs upward and outward diffusion, descent and purification, and regulates waterways. The lung is the "upper source of water." It promotes the transportation, distribution, and excretion of body fluids. The dysfunction of the lung will affect water metabolism. Its poor functioning of diffusion may result in absence of sweating and edema because fluids are unable to reach the skin, whereas its dysfunction in descent and purification may lead to inhibited urination and edema because fluids fail to be distributed to the urinary bladder. The goal of treatment is to promote lung qi to regulate the water pathway. Representative formulas include *Yue Bi Jia Zhu* Decoction (Maidservant From Yue Decoction Plus Atractylodes) and so on.

【曾经译法】 relieving lung for diuresis

【现行译法】 lifting a kettle and removing its lid; lifting kettle lid (*fig.* opening and lifting lung qi for promoting urination and defecation)

【推荐译法】 lift a kettle and remove its lid

【翻译说明】 "提壶揭盖"是比喻说法，表示开宣肺气、通利水道，以治疗癃闭、水肿等病症。为体现中医取象比类的思维方法，建议将之直译为 lift a kettle and remove its lid。


引例 Citations:


◎ 惟开展肺气，以通气化之上源，则上窍通而下窍自泄。如一壶之水，仅有在下一窍，则虽倾之而滴水不流，必为之开一上窍，则下窍遂利，此所谓下病求之于上者也。(《脏腑药式补正·膀胱部》)

（只有开宣肺气，以通调水液气化的上源，那么上窍通畅，下窍自能排泄。比如一壶的水，仅有在下一个孔，那么即便将壶倾斜也滴水不能流出；必须在上开一孔，则下窍自然通利，这就是所说的下部有病而求治于上部。）

Only when the upper source of qi transformation from water is regulated through ventilating the lung can the upper orifice become unblocked and the lower orifice (urinary bladder) excrete urine. The analogy goes like this: one cannot pour out a single drop of water even if the kettle is tilted when there is only a spout. A hole must be made in the lid of a kettle so that water can flow out. This is called treating the upper part when the lower part is diseased. (*Revision and Addition of Medicines for Zang-fu Disorders*)

◎ 肺为上焦，膀胱为下焦，上焦闭则下焦塞，如滴水之器，必上窍通而后下窍之水出焉。(《古今医案按》)

（肺在上焦，膀胱在下焦，上焦闭阻会使下焦阻塞，好像滴水的器具，必须上口通畅，然后水才能从下口流出。）

The lung is in the upper *jiao* (energizer), and the urinary bladder in the lower. The obstruction in the upper will lead to stagnation in the lower. Similar to a dripping utensil, only when the upper opening is unblocked can the water flow out of the lower opening. (*Commentaries on Ancient and Modern Case Records*) fǔdǐchōuxīn

# 釜底抽薪

Remove the Firewood from Under the Cauldron

釜底抽薪，一般比喻从根本上解决问题。中医学则用以比喻对火热亢盛之证，采用攻下的方法以清泄火热。如当伤寒传至阳明，燥热内结，阴液灼伤的情况下，紧急采用攻下方法，通便泻热，以保存阴液不被消耗殆尽，中医也称为"急下存阴法"。急下存阴法针对的病证主要有两种：一种是阳明腑热炽盛；一种是少阴热化而热传阳明，热盛阴伤。治疗多采用大承气汤。

The term is often used metaphorically to mean tackling the root of the problem. In traditional Chinese medicine, it refers to a method of purging fire in excessive fire-heat pattern. For example, when cold damage is transmitted to *yangming* meridians, dryness heat is accumulated in the body, consuming yin fluids. To preserve yin fluids, purgation is therefore used urgently to relieve constipation and heat. This method is also named "purging to preserve yin." It is primarily used for two patterns: excessive heat in *yangming fu*-organs and excessive heat damaging yin fluids due to heat of *shaoyin* transmitted to *yangming*. *Da Cheng Qi* Decoction (Major Decoction for Purging Digestive Qi) is often used.

【曾经译法】 removing burning wood from under the boiler; taking drastic measure to treat disease; taking away burning wood from under the boiler; taking the fire-wood from beneath the cauldron

【现行译法】 removing burning wood from under the boiler; taking away firewood from under the cauldron (elimination of sthenia-heat with cold and purgative drugs); taking away firewood from under the cauldron (*fig.* a method of clearing heat by purgation); taking away fire wood from under cauldron

【推荐译法】 remove the firewood from under the cauldron

【翻译说明】"釜"是一种圆底无足的炊具，类似今天使用的"锅"。译词 cauldron 指架在火上烹煮液体或食物的大锅，符合语境，而 boiler 指锅炉或汽锅，与"釜"不同。"薪"指柴火，可译为 firewood。"釜底抽薪"字面意思是指把柴火从锅底抽掉，为体现中医取象比类的思维方法，建议译为 remove the firewood from under the cauldron。

引例 Citations:

◎ 汗后不解，宜汗下兼行，加大黄乃釜底抽薪之法。(《伤寒集验》卷一)

（发汗以后病情没有缓解，应发汗、泻下同时使用，加用大黄，这就是釜底抽薪的方法。）

When a patient's symptoms are not alleviated after sweating, simultaneous use of sweating and purging therapies are necessary, and *dahuang* (*Radix et Rhizoma Rhei*, rhubarb root and rhizome) should be added. This is removing the firewood from under the cauldron. (*Collection of Experience on Cold Damage*)

◎ 三曰攻。火气郁结，大便不通，法当攻下，此釜底抽薪之法，如承气汤之类是也。(《医学心悟》卷一)

（第三为攻法，火热郁结，大便不通，治法应当用攻下，这就是釜底抽薪的方法，例如用承气汤之类。）

Purging is the third method. It should be used in the case of constipation due to fire-heat stagnation. This is removing the firewood from under the cauldron. For instance, *Cheng Qi* Decoction (Decoction for Purging Digestive Qi) is a typical formula. (*Medical Understanding*) bǔtǔ-fúhuǒ

# 补土伏火

Tonify Earth to Subdue Fire

补土伏火，是指补益脾胃、益气温阳，以治疗与脾虚相关的内生火热疾病，使元气足而阴火散，阳气复而火自安位，所谓"五行之要在中土""土厚火自敛"。若脾胃虚弱，升降运转和气血生化两大基本功能失常，可致清阳不升，阳气郁滞，湿浊郁阻，津血亏虚，相火离位等，最终使虚火上冲，临床可见发热、口疮、吐血、衄血、胃脘嘈杂等病症，治疗当补土伏火，常用方剂有补中益气汤、封髓丹、理中汤等。

The term refers to the method of tonifying the spleen and stomach and supplementing qi to warm yang to relieve endogenous fire heat due to spleen deficiency. Its purpose is to ensure sufficiency of original qi and dissipation of yin fire so that yang qi is restored and fire is back to its due place. This is what traditional Chinese medicine emphasizes: "Earth is the center among the five elements" and "when earth is thickened, fire is restrained." If the spleen and the stomach are weak, the function of ascending and descending as well as transformation of qi and blood will be affected, causing the inability of clear yang to ascend, stagnation of yang qi and turbid dampness, deficiency of body fluids and blood, ministerial fire in dislocation, and finally the flaring up of deficiency fire. Clinical manifestations include fever, mouth ulcers, hematemesis, nosebleeds, and epigastric noise. The goal of treatment is to tonify earth to subdue fire. Commonly used formulas include *Buzhong Yiqi* Decoction (Decoction for Tonifying Middle *Jiao* and Boosting Qi), *Feng Sui* Elixir (Marrow-retaining Elixir), and *Li Zhong* Decoction (Center-regulating Decoction).

【曾经译法】无

【现行译法】无

【推荐译法】tonify earth to subdue fire

【翻译说明】"补土伏火"是指通过补益脾土来达到泻火的目的，脾在五行属土；subdue 意为"制伏；控制"。"补土伏火"可译为tonify earth to subdue fire。

引例 Citations:

◎ 脾土太弱，不能伏火，火不潜藏，真阳之气外越……土薄不能伏之，即大补其土以伏火。(《医理真传》)

（脾气太弱，不能制伏阴火，火不能潜藏，真阳向外浮越……脾土虚弱不能制伏阴火，就大补脾土以制伏阴火。）

When spleen qi is too weak to control yin fire, true yang comes forth from the interior due to the failure of fire to conceal itself... When (spleen) earth is too weak to subdue fire, the aim of treatment is to tonify it to subdue fire. (*True Transmission of Medical Principles*)

◎ 火有虚实，虚火又有阴虚火炎与气（阳）虚火不安位之别，气（阳）虚火不安位之火，即是阴火，也就是补土伏火之"火"。(《读书析疑与临证得失》)

（火有虚火与实火，虚火又有阴虚火炎与气（阳）虚火不安位两种情况。气（阳）虚火不安位的火即是阴火，也就是补土伏火之"火"。）

Fire is categorized into deficiency fire and excess fire. Deficiency fire is then subdivided into fire flaring-up due to yin deficiency and fire in dislocation due to qi (yang) deficiency. The latter is called yin fire, and is the type of fire that a physician tonifies the spleen to subdue. (*Resolving Doubts in Reading and Gains and Losses in Clinical Practice*) zēngshuǐ-xíngzhōu

# 增水行舟

Increase Water to Move the Boat

日常生活经验告诉人们，河道干涸，水浅泥淤，则舟船难行。基于此生活经验，中医学将通过滋阴增液以治疗液亏便秘或血瘀的治疗方法，称为"增水行舟"。本法多用于温病高热，或吐泻、大汗、烧伤等因素导致津液大量亏耗，一方面使肠失濡润，燥屎不行，大便燥结不通。另一方面使血容量减少，血液循行滞涩不畅，而发生血瘀病变。治疗自当滋阴增液，使水涨舟行，代表方如增液汤。此法现代拓展用于血栓性疾病、尿路结石、黄疸等病证。

Daily life experience has taught us that when the river bed is dry or its water is shallow and muddy, it will be difficult for boats to travel along. Based on this, traditional Chinese medicine physicians treat constipation due to fluid deficiency or blood stasis by nourishing yin to increase fluids, which is termed "increasing water to drive the boat to move." It is mainly used to relieve large fluid loss due to high fever caused by warm diseases, or due to factors such as vomiting, diarrhea, profuse sweating, and burns. Large fluid loss deprives the intestine of the moisture it needs, causing dry stools that are difficult to pass out. It also causes reduced blood volume and blood flow obstruction, resulting in blood stasis. The goal of treatment is to nourish yin to increase fluids so that a rising tide drives the boat to move. One of the representative formulas is *Zengye* Decoction (Fluid-increasing Decoction). In modern times, this method can also be used to treat diseases such as thrombotic disorders, urinary calculi, and jaundice.

【曾经译法】 a boat floating with the upflowing tide; increase humor to move the grounded ship [move hard stool]; raising water to run ships; increasing body fluid for curing constipation

【现行译法】increasing water to make the boat going; increasing body fluid to relieve constipation; Raising Water to Run Boat; smooth sailing with water rising; increasing body fluid for curing constipation; increasing fluid to move the boat; refloating the grounded ship; a rising tide lifting traveling boats (increasing body fluid to relieve constipation); Formulas that generate fluids to promote bowel movements

【推荐译法】increase water to move the boat

【翻译说明】"增水行舟"是比喻说法，意思是通过滋阴增液以治疗液亏便秘或血瘀。为体现中医取象比类的思维方法，建议将之直译为 increase water to move the boat。


引例 Citations:


◎ 津液为火灼竭，则血行瘀滞……夫血犹舟也，津液水也。医者于此，当知增水行舟之义。(《读医随笔》)

（津液因火灼伤而虚衰，会使血液运行瘀阻不畅……血好像舟船，津液好像河水。医生遇到这种情况，应知道增水行舟的意义。）

Fluids become deficient due to scorching fire and it causes blood flow obstruction... Blood is the boat, and fluids are water. Physicians are expected to know the value of increasing water to move the boat when they come across such a disorder. (*Random Notes While Reading About Medicine*)

◎ 三者（玄参、麦冬、生地）合用作增水行舟之计，故汤名增液，但非重用不为功。(《温病条辨·中焦篇》)

（玄参、麦冬、生地三药合用，作为增水行舟的计策，因此方名增液，但不重用不能取效。）

The combined use of *xuanshen* (*Radix Scrophulariae*, figwort root), *maidong* (*Radix Ophiopogonis*, dwarf lilyturf tuber), and *shengdi* (*Radix Rehmanniae*, rehmannia root) serves to increase water to promote bowel movements, hence the name *Zengye* Decoction (Fluid-increasing Decoction). Nevertheless, no effect will be achieved unless a heavy dose is prescribed. (*Systematic Differentiation of Warm Diseases*) yǐnhuǒ-guīyuán

# 引火归原

## Guide Fire to Its Origin

引火归原，又名导龙入海，是指用温补阳气的药物，适当加入引经药，以治疗元阳浮越、肾火上升的方法。肾藏真阴而寓真阳，为水火之脏，阴阳之宅。若肾的阴阳水火平衡失调，就会出现阴虚阳浮、失制之火上升或阴寒内盛、无根之火外越的火不归原的病理状态。故本法适用于阴虚不能涵阳，或阴盛迫阳上越，导致虚火上浮、龙火上僭之证。若阴虚火浮，症见腰膝酸软，头晕耳鸣，遗精早泄，口干咽痛，两颧潮红，或面目升火，五心烦热，或午后潮热，舌红少苔或无苔，脉细数等，方用金匮肾气丸、镇阴煎等。若阴盛火浮，症见腰酸腿软，两足发冷或四肢厥逆，头晕耳鸣，大便溏薄或下利清谷，面色浮红，口舌糜烂，牙齿痛，舌质嫩红，脉虚大等，方用四逆汤、通脉四逆汤等。

The term is also known as guiding a dragon into the sea. It refers to a treatment method of restricting floating yang qi and rising kidney fire with medicines that warm and tonify yang qi and an appropriate addition of meridian guide. The kidney stores true yin (kidney yin) and true yang (kidney yang). It is the organ of water and fire and the house of yin and yang. When the balance of kidney yin and kidney yang is disrupted, pathological changes take place: yin becomes deficient, and yang floats; hence the unrestrained fire rises up. Or interior cold becomes excessive and rootless fire flares outside, that is, fire is not in its due origin. Therefore, the method of guiding fire to its origin is applicable to the case in which yin cannot contain yang due to its deficiency, or excessive yin forces yang to float upward, leading to the rise and flaring up of deficient fire. Manifestations of floating fire due to yin deficiency include the following: soreness and weakness of the lumbar region and knees, dizziness, tinnitus, seminal emission, premature ejaculation, dry mouth, sore throat, and flushing of the cheekbones; feverish sensation of the face and eyes, and feverish sensations in palms, soles, and chest; hot flushes in the afternoon, a red tongue with little or no coating, and a thin, rapid pulse. *Jingui Shenqi* Pill (Golden Cabinet's Kidney Qi Pill) or *Zhen Yin* Decoction (Decoction for Nourishing True Yin) can be used. Manifestations of floating fire due to excessive yin include soreness of the lumbar region and weak legs, cold feet or limbs, dizziness, tinnitus, loose stools with or without undigested food, red complexion, erosion of the mouth and tongue, tooth pain, a red, tender tongue, and a deficient, large pulse. *Si Ni* Decoction (Decoction for Treating Cold Extremities) or *Tongmai Si Ni* Decoction (Decoction for Invigorating the Pulse and Treating Cold Extremities) is usually prescribed.

【曾经译法】 guiding fire to its origin; letting the fire back to its origin; conducting the fire back to its origin; return fire to its source; directing fire to its source

【现行译法】 conducting the fire back to its origin; directing fire to its source/conducting fire to its origin; direct fire back to its origin; conducting fire back to its origin; Lead the fire back to its origin; return fire to its origin; conducting fire back to its source; returning fire to its origin; guiding fire to original place; leading fire to its origin; guiding fire to its origin; Guide fire to its origin

【推荐译法】 guide fire to its origin

【翻译说明】 "引火归原"的意思是引导上浮之虚火回归本源之位，直译就是 guide fire to its origin。相较于其他动词如 let，conduct，return，direct 或 lead，译词 guide 更能体现"引导；指引"之意。

引例 Citations:

◎ 此格阳虚火证也，速宜引火归原，用镇阴煎或八味地黄汤之类，则火自降而血自安矣。（《景岳全书·杂证谟》）

（这是阴盛格阳的虚火证，治疗应急速引火归原，方选镇阴煎或八味地黄汤等，就可使火自降而血自安。）

This is the deficiency-fire pattern caused by excessive yin rejecting yang. The treatment should be quickly guiding fire to its origin. Formulas such as *Zhen Yin* Decoction (Decoction for Nourishing True Yin) and *Bawei Dihuang* Decoction (*Eight-ingredient Rehmannia Decoction*) can direct fire downward and calm blood. (*Complete Works of Jingyue*)

◎ 当以辛热杂于壮水药中，导之下行，所谓引龙入海、引火归原，如八味汤之类是也。（《医学心悟》卷一）

（应该将辛热药物加入滋阴壮水药中，引导火热下行，即所说的引龙入海、引火归原，例如八味汤之类的方剂。）

Pungent hot medicines should be added to those that nourish yin and reinforce kidney water to guide fire heat downward, that is, to guide a dragon into the sea, or to guide fire to its origin. *Bawei* Decoction (Eight-ingredient Decoction) is a typical formula. (*Medical Understanding*) gānwēn chú rè

# 甘温除热

Reduce Fever with Sweet, Warm Medicines

甘温除热，即用味甘性温的药物治疗气虚发热或血虚发热的方法。此法是金元著名医家李东垣秉承《黄帝内经》"劳者温之""损者益之"之旨和张仲景《金匮要略》建中汤证等治法，结合自己的医疗经验创制而成。如气虚发热，症见身大热有汗、渴欲热饮、少气懒言，舌嫩色淡，脉虚大者，用补中益气汤。产后或劳倦内伤发热，症见肌热面赤、烦渴欲饮，舌淡红，脉洪大而虚，用当归补血汤。甘温之剂可以升阳益气，振奋脾阳，恢复脾胃健运功能，使气血生化有源，脏腑得濡，升降复常，则虚热自退。

The term refers to a treatment method of using medicines sweet in taste and warm in property to reduce fever due to qi deficiency or blood deficiency. It was created by Li Dongyuan, a well-known physician of the Jin and Yuan dynasties. Li followed the methods of "treating consumptive diseases by mild tonification" and "treating impairment by supplementing" in *Huangdi's Inner Canon of Medicine* and combined his own medical experience with the therapies such as *Jianzhong* Decoction (Center-fortifying Decoction) proposed by Zhang Zhongjing in *Essential Prescriptions of the Golden Cabinet*. Manifestations of fever due to qi deficiency include high fever with sweating, thirst and a desire for hot drinks, shallow breathing with little desire to talk, a pale, tender tongue, and a deficient, large pulse. *Buzhong Yiqi* Decoction (Decoction for Tonifying Middle *Jiao* and Boosting Qi) is used as a cure. Manifestations of postpartum fever or fever due to fatigue and internal dysfunction include fever, flushed face, restlessness, thirst and a desire for drinks, a pale red tongue, and a surging, large, deficient pulse. *Danggui Buxue* Decoction (Chinese Angelica Blood-supplementing Decoction) should be used. Sweet, warm medicines can promote yang qi, invigorate spleen yang, and restore the transportation-and-transformation function of the spleen and the stomach so that qi and blood are generated, the *zang-fu* organs are moistened, and the ascending and descending are normalized, resulting in the removal of deficiency heat.

【曾经译法】relieve high fever with drugs of sweet flavour and warm nature; eliminating severe heat with the sweet and warm; defervescence with drugs of sweet taste and warm nature; relieving high fever with drugs of sweet flavor and warm nature; relieving high fever with sweet-warm herbs; eliminate heat with warmth and sweetness; sweet and warm tastes removing fever; resolving heat with warm-sweet drugs; relieving fever with sweet and warm-natured drugs

【现行译法】relieving fever with drugs sweet in flavor and warm in nature; sweet and warm herbs relieving heat/relieving heat with sweet-warm herbs; relieving fever with sweet-warm; Eliminating heat with warmth and sweetness; defervescence with drugs of sweet taste and warm nature; relieving fever with sweet and warm-natured drugs; relieving acute case with sweet-lubricant herbs; eliminating severe heat with the sweet and warm; relieving fever with sweet and warm; relieving fever with sweet and warm medicinals; sweet-warm drugs expelling heat; eliminating high fever with herbs sweet in flavor and warm in property; eliminating heat with the sweet and warmth; Formulas that reduce fever with sweet, warm medicines

【推荐译法】reduce fever with sweet, warm medicines

【翻译说明】"甘温除热"表示用味甘性温的药物治疗气虚发热或血虚发热，这里的"热"为"发热"，建议译为 fever。2022 年发布的《世界卫生组织中医药术语国际标准》将之译为 formulas that reduce fever with sweet, warm medicines。考虑术语简洁性原则和不同语境，建议译为 reduce fever with sweet, warm medicines。

引例 Citations:

◎ 然甘温除热泻火之法施于作酸日，其酸转增，用必无功。(《寓意草》
卷四)

  (但是甘温除热泻火的治法，用于患者泛酸之时，他的泛酸加剧，
  用了肯定无效。)

However, the method of reducing fever and purging fire with sweet, warm
medicines does not work effectively when the patient has acid reflux. Instead,
reflux will be exacerbated. (*Yu Chang's Case Records and Treatments*)

◎ 医家不辨是非，便引东垣"劳倦伤脾，元气下陷，乃执甘温除热"之句，
转补壅热，至于不救矣。(《温热暑疫全书》卷四)

  (医生不辨清是非，就引用李东垣"劳倦伤脾，元气下陷，就用
  甘温除热"的观点，转而补益使热邪壅滞，以致病患无法救治。)

When a physician makes no differentiation and copies Li Dongyuan's method
of "reducing fever with sweet, warm medicines to treat sinking of original qi
due to spleen impairment by fatigue," the patient will be put in an incurable
condition because tonification may cause heat accumulation. (*Complete Treatise
on Summer-heat Disease and Epidemic Disease*)

jiāotōng xīn shèn

# 交通心肾

Coordinate the Heart and the Kidney

交通心肾，又称既济心肾、交济心肾，是指用具有滋肾阴、敛肾阳、降心火、安心神作用的方药，以滋阴潜阳，沟通心肾，治疗心肾不交证的治法。适应于心肾不交证，临床症见虚烦不寐，心悸，健忘多梦，头晕耳鸣，腰膝酸软，口燥咽干，五心烦热，潮热盗汗，便结尿黄，舌红少苔，脉细数。代表方有交泰丸、桑螵蛸散、坎离丹等。

The term is also known as keeping communication or interaction between the heart and the kidney. It refers to the method of nourishing yin and subduing yang to coordinate the heart and the kidney for the treatment of heart-kidney disharmony, using medicines that nourish kidney yin, secure kidney yang, reduce heart fire, and calm the mind. Clinical manifestations include vexation, insomnia, palpitations, forgetfulness, dreaminess, dizziness, tinnitus, soreness and weakness of the lumbar region and knees, dry mouth and throat, feverish sensations in palms, soles, and chest, tidal fever, night sweat, constipation, yellow urine, a red tongue with little coating, and a thready, rapid pulse. Representative formulas include *Jiao Tai* Pill (Pill for Balancing the Heart and the Kidney), *Sangpiaoxiao* Powder (Mantis Egg Shell Powder), and *Kan Li* Elixir (Elixir for Relieving Disharmony Between the Heart and the Kidney).

【曾经译法】 keep the heart-fire and the kidney-water in balance; keeping the heart in communication with the kidney; restoring normal coordination between the heart (fire) and the kidney (water); harmonizing the heart and kidney; promote heart-kidney interaction; promote interaction of the heart and kidney; restoring normal coordination between heart and kidney

【现行译法】 restoring normal coordination between the heart (fire) and the kidney (water); balancing heart and kidney/harmonizing heart and kidney/promoting interaction between heart and kidney; coordinating the heart and kidney; Restoring the equilibrium between the heart-kidney (note: "heart-kidney" should be revised as "heart and the kidney"); Restoring Normal Coordination between the Heart and Kidney; restoring normal coordination between heart (fire) and kidney (water); coordinating heart and kidney; keeping the heart in communication with the kidney; restoring coordination between heart and kidney; heart-kidney interaction; restoration of coordination between the heart and kidney; keeping coordination between the heart and kidney; communication between heart and kidney; coordinate the heart and kidney

【推荐译法】 coordinate the heart and the kidney

【翻译说明】 "交通心肾"中的"交通"意思是"沟通",译为 coordinate（让身体的不同部位协同工作）较妥。中医的"心""肾"不同于西医,建议统一在前面加定冠词, kidney 用单数形式。

引例 Citations:

◎ 交通心肾,菖蒲、远志、莲子等不可少。(《医碥》卷四)

  (交通心肾法,不能缺少菖蒲、远志、莲子等药。)

Medicines such as *changpu* (*Rhizoma Acori Tatarinowii*, grassleaf sweetflag rhizome), *yuanzhi* (*Radix Polygalae*, thin-leaf milkwort root), and *lianzi* (*Semen Nelumbinis*, lotus seed) are essential to formulas for coordinating the heart and the kidney. (*Stepping Stones for Medicine*)

◎ 惊劳失志,总由心肾不交……故以茯神、远志交通心肾。(《孙真人千金方衍义》卷十四)

（惊恐劳累，神志恍惚，总体由于心肾不交导致……因此，用茯神、远志交通心肾。）

Fright, fatigue, and trance are mainly caused by heart-kidney disharmony...
Hence, *fushen* (*Sclerotium Poriae Pararadicis*, Indian bread with hostwood)
and *yuanzhi* (*Radix Polygalae*, thin-leaf milkwort root) are used to coordinate
the two organs. (*Annotations and Elaborations on Sun Simiao's "Essential
Prescriptions Worth a Thousand Pieces of Gold"*)

yíjīng biànqì

# 移精变气

## Shift Attention and Change Qi

移精变气，是指通过语言、行为等手段移转或分散患者异常的精神意念活动指向，以缓解或消除由于精神、情志因素所引起的疾病的一种心理疗法。常用的移精变气方法有两类：一是精神转移法，即将患者的精神、意念活动从焦虑、抑郁转移或分散至其他方面，以缓解或消除因过分关注内心冲突和不良情绪所致的躯体不适形成的强化性病态条件反射及病态行为。二是情志导引法，即通过指导患者进行呼吸吐纳锻炼，或配合一些动作，引导和控制患者的精神、意念活动，达到移精变气的治疗目的。情志导引法最基本的要领为调心（意念控制）、调气（呼吸锻炼）和调身（姿势调整）合一。

The term refers to a psychotherapy that shifts or diverts a patient's attention away from mental and emotional abnormalities by means of language and behavior to alleviate or eliminate disorders caused by mental or emotional factors. It encompasses two common types: diversion of attention and *Daoyin* of emotions. The former refers to changing or diverting aspects of a patient's mental activity away from anxiety and depression to relieve or eliminate intensive pathological reflexes and behaviors that are caused by physical discomforts due to excessive attention to internal conflicts and negative emotions. The latter is a method to instruct patients to practice inhaling and exhaling (Daoist breathing techniques), along with certain physical movements, to guide and control their mental and emotional activities for the purpose of shifting attention and changing qi. Its essential components are regulation of the mind (mind control), regulation of breathing (breathing exercise), and regulation of posture (posture adjustment). The three are integrated into a whole.

【曾经译法】guided mental concentration; deviated attention

【现行译法】shifting the essence and changing qi; regulating the vital energy by shifting patient's attention; moving the essence and changing the qi

【推荐译法】shift attention and change qi

【翻译说明】"移精变气"指转移、改变患者的精神状态，其中"精"指人的思想、精神；"气"指气机。"移"和"变"意思近似。译词 deviate 意为"背离；偏离"，语义不符。为照顾回译性，建议将"移精变气"译为 shift attention and change qi。

引例 Citations:

◎ 黄帝问曰：余闻古之治病，惟其移精变气，可祝由而已。(《素问·移精变气论》)

（黄帝问道：我听说古时治病，只是改变患者的思想精神，用符咒和语言祈祷治病的方法就可以治愈。）

Huangdi (Yellow Emperor) asked: "I heard that in ancient times, healing can be achieved by simply shifting a patient's attention and changing their qi with the method of *zhuyou* (a form of psychotherapy in traditional Chinese medicine)." (*Plain Conversation*)

◎ 是以有病以祝为由，移精变气去之，无假于针药也。(《太素》卷十九)

（所以用符咒和语言祈祷治病的方法，改变患者的思想精神，不用借助于针刺、药物。）

Therefore, *zhuyou* therapy, rather than needles and medicines, is used to shift a patient's attention and change qi . (*Grand Simplicity*)

shùnqíng cóngyù

# 顺情从欲

## Satisfy Needs and Wants

顺情从欲法，又称顺意疗法，是通过满足患者平凡的意愿、感情和生理需要，以达排解心理障碍的一种心理治疗方法。此法适用于因情思不遂所致的郁证、相思病、饥饿哭啼、幼儿数日内啼哭不止、肿瘤以及其他多种心身疾病的心理治疗。采用本法治疗疾病，首先要探究患者真正的意念欲望所在。其次，医生还要耐心启发患者，采取其易于接受的方法，得到患者的充分理解和合作，患者才能将隐曲深沉的心里话说出来。对于一些无法很好地用语言沟通的患者，医生需要通过察言观色，向其身边人详细询问了解，掌握患者真正的需求。

The term, also known as submission therapy, refers to a type of psychotherapy that aims to relieve mental disorders by satisfying the common wishes as well as the emotional and physiological needs of patients. It can be used to treat a variety of psychosomatic disorders such as depression, lovesickness, hunger cry, children crying for several days, and tumors caused by emotional upsets. Before using this therapy, the physician should first explore the real needs and wants of patients. Next, the physician is expected to inquire and elicit in a patient and approachable manner to gain a full understanding and cooperation of patients so that they can reveal their inner thoughts and struggles. For patients unable to communicate well with words, the physician needs to understand their real needs by observing what they say and do and by asking people around them for details.

【曾经译法】 无

【现行译法】 submission therapy

【推荐译法】 satisfy needs and wants

【翻译说明】 "顺情从欲"简而言之就是满足患者的需求和愿望，"顺"和
"从"意思相近，建议译为 satisfy needs and wants。

引例 Citations:

◎ 未有逆而能治之也，夫惟顺而已矣。顺者，非独阴阳脉论，气之逆顺也，百姓人民皆欲顺其志也。(《灵枢·师传》)

（从来没有用逆行的方法能治理好的，只有采取顺行的方法。所谓顺，不仅是指阴阳经脉营卫之气的顺逆，对待人民百姓，也要顺着他们的意愿。）

No success can be achieved if administration goes against norms. It is only through such an approach that complies with norms can a cure become possible. Compliance refers not only to the fact that qi of yin, yang, meridians, collaterals, nutrient, and defense should travel in accordance with norms, but also to the fact that governance should be in accordance with the expectations of all people in a country. (*Miraculous Pivot*)

◎ 因病人之义而用之奈何？如病人喜食寒，即以寒物投之，病人喜食热，即以热物投之也。随病人之性，而加以顺性之方，则不违而得大益。(《石室秘录》卷五)

（顺从患者意愿而用药怎样？例如，患者喜欢进食寒凉，就给他寒凉之品；患者喜欢进食热物，就给他温热之品。随着患者性情，而使用顺从其性的方剂，就不会违背其意愿而获得较大的效益。）

How about prescribing medicines according to a patient's wishes? For instance, if a patient prefers cold-natured food, give him/her cool- or cold-natured medicines; if a patient loves hot-natured food, give him/her warm- or hot-natured medicines. When a physician takes the needs of a patient into consideration and uses a prescription that does not go against the patient's wants, greater benefits can be obtained. (*Secret Records in a Stone Room*) mùyù dá zhī

# 木郁达之

Treat Wood Stagnation by Dredging

木郁达之，语出《素问·六元正纪大论》，是指对各种肝郁气滞之证，疏肝理气解郁，使郁结的气机畅达、肝脏疏泄条达的功能本性恢复正常的治疗方法。肝喜条达而恶抑郁，外感邪气，内伤情志，脏气自损等皆可作用于肝而致郁。"木郁"病证范围较广，从病性的角度而言，朱丹溪创六郁之说，创制越鞠丸治疗气、湿、火、痰、血、食诸郁。从病位的角度而言，肝气亢逆不制，气机升降失调，则可产生克脾、犯胃、冲心、迫肺等多种病证，代表方有柴胡疏肝散、逍遥散等，精神疏导也是重要的治疗措施。

The term is derived from *Plain Conversation* ("Significant Discussions on the Changing Principles of Six Qi"). It refers to a treatment approach that aims to soothe the liver (wood) and regulate qi to relieve various liver qi stagnation so that the free flow of qi can be restored. The liver likes free will and hates to be depressed. Liver qi stagnation occurs when the liver is affected by exogenous pathogenic qi, emotional disorders, or the self-impairment of visceral qi. "Liver-qi stagnation pattern" encompasses a wide range of syndromes. In terms of disease nature, Zhu Danxi created the theory of "six stagnations" and created *Yueju* Pill (Constraint-resolving Pill) to treat the stagnation of qi, dampness, fire, phlegm, blood, and food. In terms of disease location, when liver qi is too hyperactive to be restrained, disordered activity of qi occurs in ascending and descending, resulting in a variety of disorders of the spleen, stomach, heart, and lung. Representative formulas include *Chaihu Shugan* Powder (Bupleurum Liver-soothing Powder) and *Xiaoyao* Powder (Free Wanderer Powder). Besides, psychological counseling is also an important treatment method.

【曾经译法】 facilitating the stagnant wood; stagnated liver-energy (wood) should be released; depressed wood is treated by outthrust; facilitating hepatic stagnation

【现行译法】treating depression of the liver (wood) by soothing method; wood depression can be treated by relief therapy/liver depression can be treated by relief therapy; mollify the liver (wood) if it is depressed; depression of liver (wood) which should be relieved; Depressed liver (wood) needs to be mollified; facilitating the stagnant wood; wood-depression being treated by soothing therapy; mollify the liver (wood) if it is depressed

【推荐译法】treat wood stagnation by dredging

【翻译说明】"木郁"指肝郁气滞之证，直译为 wood stagnation，常意译为 liver-qi stagnation。译词 stagnation 多表示"停滞；淤滞"。"达"指"疏通、畅达"，可译为 dredge（疏浚，清淤）。以往译法中的 facilitate 多表示"促进；促使"，release 多表示"释放；松开；解除；公开"，outthrust 表示"（使）突出；（使）伸出"，soothing 多表示"安慰；缓解；缓和"，relieve 多表示"解除；减轻；缓和"，mollify 常表示"安抚；使平静"。"木郁达之"指用疏通的方法治疗肝郁气滞之证，考虑到类似术语结构翻译的一致性，可译为 treat wood stagnation by dredging，但"木郁"二字往往译为 liver-qi stagnation。

引例 Citations:

◎《内经》曰木郁达之，木郁者，肝郁也；达者，条达、通达之谓也。（《医旨绪余》卷上）

（《黄帝内经》说：木郁达之。木郁，即是肝郁；达，即条达、通达之义。）

*Huangdi's Inner Canon of Medicine* states: "*Muyu* (木郁) *da* (达) *zhi* (之)." *Muyu*, literally meaning "wood stagnation", refers to liver-qi stagnation; *da*

means "to dredge something for a smooth flow." (*Remnants of Medical Decree*)

◎ 木郁达之，达者，通畅之谓，或升发，或轻散，或宣越，皆达之之法，不可以吐为达也。(《济阳纲目》卷二十七)

（木郁达之，达有疏通、畅达之义，或者升发，或者轻散，或者宣越，都是使气机畅达的方法，不能简单地认为涌吐就是畅达气机。）

Treat liver-qi stagnation by dredging. A variety of methods can contribute to the unblocked flow of qi, for instance, lifting, dissipating, and diffusing. One cannot simply take vomiting as the sole method to unblock qi flow. (*Guide to Saving Yang*) huǒyù fā zhī

# 火郁发之

## Treat Fire Stagnation by Expelling

火郁发之，语出《素问·六元正纪大论》，是指邪热郁伏不出，用宣散、升举、轻扬、疏通等法治疗的一种方法。火郁，是指火热之邪郁闭，包括外感六淫之邪侵袭化火生热，郁伏不得出，或内生火热郁闭体内。临床表现复杂多样，其共同特征为具有口苦咽干，渴喜冷饮，少汗，小便黄赤，大便燥结，舌红苔黄，脉沉数有力等里热证，同时可见四肢逆冷、喜暖恶冷等外寒假象。"发"有发散、宣扬、疏导、启闭之义，即用清热泻火药的同时，加入少许辛温或辛凉之品以发散、宣畅气机，使郁积之火热发越透达而出。如四逆散中的柴胡，麻杏石甘汤中的麻黄，仙方活命饮中的防风、白芷等，都有"火郁发之"之义。

The term is derived from *Plain Conversation* ("Significant Discussions on the Changing Principles of Six Qi"). It refers to a treatment approach that aims to remove the fire-heat stagnation by dispersing, lifting, clearing, and dredging. Fire stagnation means the stagnation of pathogenic fire heat, including the transformed fire due to the invasion of six pathogenic factors and the internal heat accumulated in the body. Though clinical manifestations are complex and varied, common characteristics of its interior-heat pattern include bitter mouth, dry throat, thirst for cold drinks, little sweating, dark yellow urine, dry stools, a red tongue with yellow coating, and a deep, rapid, forceful pulse. At the same time, there may be false manifestations of exterior cold such as cold limbs, a preference for warmth, and an aversion to coldness. "Expelling" encompasses a range of meanings, including dispersing, clearing, dredging, and opening. A few pungent-warm or pungent-cool medicines are added to the prescriptions of clearing heat and purging fire to dissipate and promote the flow of qi so that the accumulated fire heat can be removed. For example, *Chaihu* (*Radix Bupleuri*, Chinese thorowax root) in *Si Ni* Powder (Powder for Treating Cold Extremities), *mahuang* (*Herba Ephedrae*, ephedra) in *Ma*

*Xing Shi Gan* Decoction (Ephedra, Apricot Kernel, Gypsum, and Licorice Decoction), *Fangfeng* (*Radix Saposhnokoviae*, divaricate saposhnikovia root) and *Baizhi* (*Radix Angelicae Dahuricae*, angelica root) in *Xianfang Huoming* Drink (Immortal Formula Life-giving Drink) are used to expel fire stagnation.

【曾经译法】 dissipating excessive fire stagnation; Pathogenic heat smoldering in the body should be treated with expellants or repellents; fire depression is treated by effusion; fire stagnation requiring dissipation

【现行译法】 expelling fire stagnancy; fire-stagnation should be dissipated; expel the fire if it is accumulated; Dispersing stagnant fire; dissipating excessive stagnation; fire stagnation requiring dissipation; expel the fire if it is accumulated; Formulas that effuse stagnant fire/ heat

【推荐译法】 treat fire stagnation by expelling

【翻译说明】 "火郁发之" 指用升发、轻散、宣越等方法治疗火郁之证。 "火郁" 译为 fire stagnation。 "发" 字蕴含多义，此处建议 译为宽泛的 expelling（排出；喷出；祛除）。以往译法中的 dissipate 多表示 "消散；驱散"；effuse 多表示 "分泌；泻出"； disperse 多表示 "分散；疏散；散布；传播"。


引例 Citations:


◎ 火郁发之，发者，升散之谓，或汗解，或升举，或从治，皆发之之法， 不可以汗为发也。（《济阳纲目》卷二十七）

（火郁发之，发者，意谓升散，或者汗解，或者升举，或者从治， 都属于火郁发之的方法，不能简单地认为发汗就是发越火气。）

Treat fire stagnation by expelling. The therapeutic method of sweating, lifting, or paradoxical treatment are all the methods to expel fire stagnation. One can't simply take sweating as the sole method. (*Guide to Saving Yang*)

◎ 火郁发之者，升而散之，得汗而解，此非治火，乃治火之郁也，若火非郁，则不宜升发矣。(《素问释义·六元正纪大论》)

(火郁发之者，即采用升散的方法，使汗出而解，这并不是治火，而是治火气抑郁。假如火气没有抑郁，就不能用升发的方法。)

Treat fire stagnation by expelling. By means of lifting and dispersing, sweating is induced to dissipate fire stagnation. It targets at removing the stagnation of fire, not fire itself. Lifting-and-dispersing method cannot be used if there is no stagnation. (*Interpretation of "Plain Conversation"*) tǔyù duó zhī

# 土郁夺之

## Treat Earth Stagnation by Removing

　　土郁夺之，语出《素问·六元正纪大论》，指对湿邪郁阻中焦脾胃，壅滞不通，用各种除湿之法治疗的一种方法。如湿热郁阻中焦，而见腹痛腹胀，大便稀薄而热臭，舌苔黄腻，可用苦寒以燥湿清热治之，代表方如王氏连朴饮；寒湿郁滞而见胸闷，恶心呕吐，腹胀，大便清稀，可用芳香苦温化湿治之，代表方如平胃散、藿香正气散、三仁汤等。

The term is derived from *Plain Conversation* ("Significant Discussions on the Changing Principles of Six Qi"). It refers to a treatment approach that aims to use various methods to remove the dampness that stagnates in the middle *jiao* (middle energizer, i.e., spleen and stomach) and obstructs the flow of qi. When dampness heat accumulates in the middle *jiao*, there are manifestations of abdominal pain and distention, loose and smelly stools, and a yellow, greasy tongue coating. Medicines bitter in taste and cold in property are used to eliminate dampness and heat. *Wang's Lian Pu* Drink (Wang's Coptis and Officinal Magnolia Bark Drink) is one of the representative formulas. In the case of cold-dampness stagnation, there are manifestations of chest tightness, nausea, vomiting, abdominal distention, and loose stools. Fragrant, bitter, and warm-natured medicines are used to transform dampness. Representative formulas include *Ping Wei* Powder (Stomach-Calming Powder), *Huoxiang Zhengqi* Powder (Agastache Qi-correcting Powder), and *San Ren* Decoction (Three Kernels Decoction).

【曾经译法】 eliminating the stagnant earth; Dampness accumulated in the spleen (earth) should be removed; Earth stagnancy is treated by removing dampness; depressed earth is treated by despoliation; gastro-stagnation requiring expelling therapy; depressed earth is treated by retrenchment

【现行译法】 removing damp accumulated in the spleen (earth); spleen depression should be treated by eliminating dampness; remove the damp if it is accumulated in the spleen (earth); dampness accumulated in spleen (earth) which should be removed; eliminating the stagnant earth; removing accumulated dampness from the spleen; depression being removed from earth (spleen and stomach); remove dampness if it is accumulated in the spleen (earth)

【推荐译法】 treat earth stagnation by removing

【翻译说明】 "土郁夺之"指用各种祛湿的方法治疗脾气壅滞不通。"土郁"指脾气郁滞，直译为 earth stagnation，意译为 spleen-qi stagnation；"夺"为夺取，译为 remove（拿走；夺走）。译词 eliminate 强调去除自己不想要、不需要的东西；despoliation 表示"掠夺，抢劫"；expelling 表示"排出；喷出；祛除"；retrenchment 表示"紧缩；消减（开支）"。建议将"土郁夺之"译为 treat earth stagnation by removing，或根据上下文译为 treat spleen-qi stagnation by removing。


引例 Citations:


◎ 土郁夺之，夺者，攘取之谓，或攻下，或劫而衰之，皆夺之之法，不可以下为夺也。（《济阳纲目》卷二十七）

（土郁夺之，夺者，意谓夺取，或者攻下，或者强取而使邪气衰减，都是夺去壅滞的方法，不能简单地认为攻下就是夺去土气壅滞。）


Treat earth stagnation by removing. Methods of purging and taking by force are used to relieve pathogenic factors and remove spleen-qi stagnation. One can't simply take purging as the sole method. (*Guide to Saving Yang*)

◎ 土郁夺之，土郁者，脾郁也；夺者，攘夺之谓也。土性贵燥，惟燥乃能运化精微而致各脏也。（《医旨绪余》卷上）

（土郁夺之，土郁，即脾气抑郁；夺者，意谓劫夺。土性喜燥，只有燥才能运化精微而转输到各脏腑。）

Treat earth stagnation by removing. Earth stagnation refers to spleen-qi depression. Removing means taking away by force. The spleen pertains to earth, which likes dryness. Only dryness can facilitate transformation and transport essence to all *zang-fu* organs. (*Remnants of Medical Decree*) jīnyù xiè zhī

# 金郁泄之

Treat Metal Stagnation by Dredging

金郁泄之，语出《素问·六元正纪大论》，指对各种原因导致的肺气郁闭不利之证，采用疏利气机以宣通肺气的治疗方法。如肺气不宣，则水道不畅，以致咳嗽气喘，水肿，小便不利，治以宣通肺气之法，方如葶苈大枣泻肺汤；热邪壅肺，肺失肃降，腑气不通，以致喘促不宁，大便秘结，脉实大，治以宣肺通腑之法，方如宣白承气汤等。

The term is derived from *Plain Conversation* ("Significant Discussions on the Changing Principles of Six Qi"). It refers to a treatment approach that aims to relieve lung-qi stagnation due to various causes by smoothing qi movement and promoting lung-qi circulation. If lung qi fails to disperse, obstruction in water pathways will occur, causing cough, panting, edema, and inhibited urination. The therapy for dispersing and ventilating lung qi is used, using formulas such as *Tingli Dazao Xiefei* Decoction (Descurainiae and Jujube Lung-purging Decoction). If pathogenic heat accumulates in the lung, the lung will fail to govern descent and purification, and qi stagnation in the *fu*-organs may occur, causing dyspnea, constipation, and an excess, large pulse. The therapy for dispersing lung qi and purging the *fu*-organs is used, such as *Xuan Bai Cheng Qi* Decoction (Decoction for Descending Lung-qi and Purging Digestive Qi).

【曾经译法】 purging the stagnant gold (note: "gold" should be revised as "metal"); depressed metal is treated by discharge; drainage for pulmonary depression; depressed metal is treated by drainage

【现行译法】 treating lung-qi stagnancy by elimination or regulation; pulmonary stagnation should be relieved; purge the lung (metal) if it is obstructed; purging the stagnant gold (note: "gold" should be revised as "metal")

【推荐译法】 treat metal stagnation by dredging

【翻译说明】"金"指五行中的"金"，对应 metal，不能译为 gold（黄金）。"金郁"指肺气郁滞，直译为 metal stagnation，意译为 lung-qi stagnation。"泄"译为 dredge（清淤，疏浚，疏通），表示宣泄疏利。"金郁泄之"可译为 treat metal stagnation by dredging，或根据上下文，译为 treat lung-qi stagnation by dredging。

引例 Citations:

◎ 金郁泄之，泄者，露去之谓，或渗泄利小便，或疏通其气，皆泄之之法，不可以利为泄也。（《济阳纲目》卷二十七）

（金郁泄之，泄者，意谓泄露去除，或者渗泄利小便，或者疏通气机，都是宣泄疏利的方法，不能简单地认为利小便就是宣泄肺气郁滞。）

Treat metal stagnation by dredging. Dredging means removing or getting rid of something. Draining, promoting urination, or smoothing qi movement are all methods to relieve lung-qi stagnation. One can't simply take promoting urination as the sole method. (*Guide to Saving Yang*)

◎ 金郁泄之，金郁者，肺郁也；泄者，疏泄之谓也。（《医旨绪余》卷上）

（金郁泄之，金郁者，意谓肺气郁滞；泄者，意谓疏泄。）

As for the term *jinyu* (金郁) *xie* (泄) *zhi* (之), *jinyu*, literally "metal stagnation", refers to lung-qi stagnation; *xie* means promoting qi flow. (*Remnants of Medical Decree*) shuǐyù zhé zhī

# 水郁折之

Treat Water Stagnation by Draining

水郁折之，语出《素问·六元正纪大论》，是指针对水寒之气盛行，郁滞于内，导致水肿、胀满、痹痛等病证，调理相关脏腑功能，以温阳蠲寒除湿利水的治法。具体如张仲景用苓桂枣甘汤治水饮奔豚证，用五苓散治太阳蓄水证，用真武汤治阳虚水泛证，或用乌头汤、白术附子汤治疗寒痹骨痛等，均属此法。

The term is derived from *Plain Conversation* ("Significant Discussions on the Changing Principles of Six Qi"). It refers to a treatment approach that aims to warm yang, eliminate cold and dampness, and promote urination by regulating the functions of related *zang-fu* organs. When water-cold is excessive and accumulates in the body, there will be such manifestations as edema, sensation of fullness, and pain caused by *bi* (impediment). Examples of this treatment method are as follows. Zhang Zhongjing used *Ling Gui Zao Gan* Decoction (Poria, Cinnamon, Dates, and Licorice Decoction) to treat running-piglet pattern caused by fluid retention, *Wu Ling* Powder (Five-ingredient Powder with Poria) to treat *taiyang* water-retention pattern, *Zhen Wu* Decoction (True Warrior Decoction) to treat yang deficiency and water-flooding pattern, and used *Wutou* Decoction (Aconite Decoction) and *Baizhu Fuzi* Decoction (White Atractylodes and Aconite Decoction) to treat bone pain caused by cold impediment.

【曾经译法】 draining the stagnant water; retention of fluid to be treated with draining method; Water stagnancy is treated by draining; depressed water is treated by regulation; regulating fluid stagnation

【现行译法】 treating retention of fluid with draining method; water stagnation should be treated by drainage; drain water if it is retained; draining the stagnant water; retained fluid removed by drainage; water depression being treated by drainage; drain the kidney if water is retained

【推荐译法】treat water stagnation by draining

【翻译说明】"水郁折之"指用疏通驱逐的方法治疗水气郁滞。"水郁"用
water stagnation 表示。译词 drain 表示"排水;(使)流走,
流出"。建议将"水郁折之"译为 treat water stagnation by
draining。

引例 Citations:

◎ 水郁折之, 折者, 曲激之谓, 或制御, 或伐挫, 或渐杀, 其势皆折之
之法, 不可以抑为折也。(《济阳纲目》卷二十七)

　　(水郁折之, 折者, 意谓弯曲冲激, 或者统治掌控, 或者砍伐摧
　　折, 或者逐渐消减, 其作用都是驱逐水气的方法, 不能简单地认
　　为抑制就是驱逐水气。)

As for the term *shuiyu* (水郁, water stagnation) *zhe* (折) *zhi* (之, it), *zhe* has a
number of meanings: bending, flushing, ruling, cutting, breaking, and reducing.
All are methods to drain water retention. One cannot simply take restraining as
the sole method. (*Guide to Saving Yang*)

◎ 水郁折之, 水郁者, 肾郁也; 折者, 决折之谓也。(《医旨绪余》卷上)

　　(水郁折之, 水郁者, 肾水郁滞; 折者, 疏通驱逐之义。)

For *shuiyu* (水郁) *zhe* (折) *zhi* (之), *shuiyu* refers to kidney-water stagnation; *zhe*
means removal by draining. (*Remnants of Medical Decree*)

shàng bìng zhì xià

# 上病治下

Treat the Lower for the Upper

上病治下，又称上病下取，指症状表现在人体上部，但疾病的病位却在下部，或根据人体上下脏腑经脉之间的联系，上部病症从下部来治疗的一种方法。疾病病位所在之本与临床表现之象，既可能一致，也可能相反。若表现一致，如病位在上，临床表现也在上，或病位在下，临床表现亦在下，那么治疗时病在上取之上，病在下取之下。否则，病位所在之本与临床表现之象不一致，如病位在上而表现于下，或病位在下而表现于上，治疗则当"病在上，取之下；病在下，取之上"（《素问·五常政大论》）。

The term, also known as "treating a disease in the upper by targeting at the lower," refers to a treatment approach that aims to cure a disease in the upper part of the body by treating the lower part. Signs and symptoms occur in the upper part of the body, but the disease location is identified in the lower part. Alternatively, the disorder in the upper part is treated by needling the acupoints in the lower part in accordance with the connections of *zang-fu* organs, meridians, and collaterals. Disease location can be in accordance with or contrary to clinical manifestations. When they are aligned, that is, both disease location and clinical manifestations are in the upper part, or both are in the lower part, treat the disease in the upper by targeting at the upper or treat the disease in the lower by targeting at the lower. Otherwise, when they are opposite, treat the disease in the upper by targeting at the lower or treat the disease in the lower by targeting at the upper. It is often shortened to "treating the lower for the upper; treating the upper for the lower," as is stated in *Plain Conversation* ("Significant Discussions on the Administration of Five-motions").

【曾经译法】 treat the diseases in the upper portion by managing the lower portion; treating the lower part for diseases of the upper; treating diseases in the upper part by managing the lower; treating the lower to cure the diseases in the upper; treating upper body disease through the lower body; needling the lower for the upper; treating diseases in upper part by managing the lower; treat upper body disease through the lower body

【现行译法】 treating disease in the upper part of the body by managing the lower; treating the lower to cure the upper disease; treating the lower for the upper; Treating upper body disease through the lower body; treating diseases in upper part by managing the lower; treating the lower part for diseases of the upper; treating lower portion for upper disorder; needling applied to the lower body to treat upper disorders

【推荐译法】 treat the lower for the upper

【翻译说明】 "上病治下"指病位在下部而表现于上部，就从下部来治疗。治疗手法不只是针刺治疗（needling），因此，建议选择 treat 翻译"治"。为照顾术语简洁性，"上病治下"可译为 treat the lower for the upper。


引例 Citations:


◎ 久嗽为喘，而气泄于上者，宜固其肺，尤宜急固其肾，所谓上病下取也。（《成方切用》卷二）

（日久咳嗽发展为喘证，肺气泄越于上者，治疗应使肺气充足，尤其应迅速使肾气充足，此即所说的病在上而取下部治疗。）

If prolonged cough develops into the pattern of asthma and lung qi ascends to the upper part, the treatment should be ensuring the sufficiency of lung qi. Especially kidney qi should be strengthened. This is treating the lower for the upper. (*Effective Use of Established Formulas*)

◎ 症本深思远虑，扰动五志之阳，化作龙雷之火，消烁脏阴营液，经旨有煎厥症名，近于此也，上病下取，滋苗灌根实下为主。(《问斋医案》卷五)

（病症由于过度思虑，扰动五脏阳气，化为亢盛的病理之火，消灼五脏阴液，《黄帝内经》有"煎厥"的病名，与此相近，病在上而治在下，滋养禾苗以灌溉根部补养下部为主。）

Due to excessive thinking, yang qi of the five *zang*-organs is disrupted and transformed into hyperactive pathological fire, which boils the yin fluids of the five *zang*-organs. It is similar to "scorching syncope" stated in *Huangdi's Inner Canon of Medicine*. The disease is located in the upper part, but the lower part is treated instead, like nourishing a plant by delivering water and nutrients to its root and lower part. (*Wenzhai's Case Records*) xià bìng zhì shàng

# 下病治上

Treat the Upper for the Lower

　　下病治上，又称下病上取，指症状表现在人体下部，但疾病的病位却在上部，或根据人体上下脏腑经脉之间的联系，下部病症从上部来治疗的一种方法。如足痛足肿，无力虚软，臁疮红肿，属中气下陷，湿热下流，用补中益气升提之；肺热所致的下肢痿症，宜清肺热；治泄泻，用实脾利水之剂不效，亦用升提；治尿血，用凉血利水不效，宜清心莲子饮清心；治大便下血，属脾虚不能摄血，宜用六君子加炮姜等。其他如脱肛、中气下陷可艾灸百会；肺气不宣而引起的小便不利可用宣通肺气等，均为下病治上之例。

The term, also known as "treating a disease in the lower by targeting at the upper," refers to a treatment approach that aims to cure a disease in the lower part of the body by treating the upper part. Signs and symptoms occur in the lower part of the body, but the disease location is identified in the upper part. Alternatively, the disorder in the lower part of the body is treated by needling acupoints in the upper part in accordance with the connections of *zang-fu* organs, meridians, and collaterals. The following are examples of treating the upper for the lower. For spleen-qi sinking and dampness heat flowing downward characterized by foot pain and swelling, weakness, and red, swelling shank sores, qi of the spleen and stomach should be tonified. For flaccidity of lower limbs caused by lung heat, lung heat should be cleared. To treat diarrhea, when the prescription of strengthening the spleen and draining dampness does not work well, medicines for lifting and ascending should be prescribed. To treat blood urination, when the prescription of cooling blood and promoting urination does not work well, *Qingxin Lianzi* Drink (Heart-clearing Lotus Seed Drink) should be used to clear heat in the heart. To treat blood stools caused by deficient spleen failing to control blood, *Liu Junzi* Decoction (Decoction of Six Noble Ingredients) should be used in combination with processed ginger. In the case of prolapse of anus and sinking of spleen-stomach qi, moxa therapy can be performed on *Baihui* acupoint (GV20). Inhibited urination caused by lung qi failing to disperse can be treated by ventilating lung qi.

【曾经译法】 treat the diseases in the lower portion by managing the upper portion; treating the upper part for diseases of the lower; treating diseases of the lower part of the body by needling points on the upper part of the body; treating diseases in the lower by needling points in the upper; treating lower body disease through the upper body; needling the upper for the lower; treat lower body disease through the upper body

【现行译法】 treating diseases of the lower part of the body by managing the upper; needling acupoints in the upper to treat disease in the lower; treating the upper for the lower; Treating lower body disease through the upper body; selecting the upper to treat the lower/treating disease of lower part of body by needling points on the upper; treating the upper part for diseases of the lower; treating upper portion for lower disorder; treating diseases in the lower part of the body by needling acupoints in the upper; treating lower disease by needling the upper

【推荐译法】 treat the upper for the lower

【翻译说明】 "下病治上"指病位在上部而表现于下部，就从上部来治疗。治疗手法不只是针刺治疗（needling），因此，建议选择用 treat 翻译"治"。为照顾术语简洁性，"下病治上"可译为 treat the upper for the lower。

引例 Citations:

◎ 欲降先升，欲升先降，上病治下，下病治上之类，决非治一切器物可以比拟也。（《医学一贯》）

（想降而先升，想升而先降，上病治下，下病治上之类，绝不是治理所有器具可以比拟的。）

Ascending for the purpose of descending, descending for the purpose of ascending, treating the lower for the upper, and treating the upper for the lower—managing all other things are by no means compared to these treatment strategies. (*Consistent Medical Principles*)

◎ 久遗成淋，而精脱于下者，宜固其肾，尤宜兼固其气，所谓下病上取也。（《成方切用》卷二）

（遗尿日久而形成淋证，精气脱失于下，应该使肾气充足，尤其应同时巩固上焦之气使之充足，此即所说的病在下而取上部治疗。）

Strangury due to prolonged enuresis causes the loss of essential qi in the lower part. Kidney qi should be strengthened. Especially the qi of the upper *jiao* (energizer) should be consolidated to achieve sufficiency. This is treating the upper for the lower. (*Effective Use of Established Formulas*) yòng hán yuǎn hán

# 用寒远寒

Avoid Cold-property Medicines in the Cold Season

　　用寒远寒，中医因时制宜用药思路之一，即冬季阴盛阳弱，病易化寒伤阳，当慎用寒药，以免更伤其阳。人体受自然界影响，其生理阴阳趋向是"春夏则阳气多而阴气少，秋冬则阴气盛而阳气衰"（《素问·厥论》）。人体在秋冬阴寒之季，病变多为寒邪伤阳，机体阴阳失调而呈现的是阴气盛而阳气衰。因此，临床用药之时，应注意寒冷季节慎用大寒的药物。

The term refers to the principle of using medicines according to time in traditional Chinese medicine. In wintertime, yin is predominant and yang is weak. It is easy for diseases to transform into cold and impair yang, so cold-property medicines should be used with caution to avoid further impairment of yang qi. Influenced by natural environment, the human body is apt to have "more yang and less yin in spring and summer, and more yin and less yang in autumn and winter" (*Plain Conversation*, "Syncope"). In the cool autumn and cold winter, disorders are mainly caused by pathogenic cold impairing yang, and yin-yang disharmony is manifested by yin excess and yang deficiency in the human body. Therefore, in clinical practice, medicines with great cold property should be cautiously used during the cold season.

【曾经译法】无

【现行译法】avoiding drugs of cool or cold nature in cold climate; avoiding using cold medicinals in winter; avoiding using cold-propertied (note: "cold-propertied" should be revised as "cold-property") medicines in cold weather

【推荐译法】avoid cold-property medicines in the cold season

【翻译说明】"用寒远寒"中第一个"寒"指药性寒凉，译为 cold-property medicines；第二个"寒"指寒冷季节，译为 the cold season。

"远"指"远离；避开"，译为 avoid。"用寒远寒"可译为 avoid cold-property medicines in the cold season。

引例 Citations:

◎ 用寒远寒，用凉远凉，用温远温，用热远热，食宜同法。(《素问·六元正纪大论》)

（用寒药时要避开寒冷的气候，用凉药时要避开清凉的气候，用温药时要避开温暖的气候，用热药时要避开炎热的气候，饮食也应该遵循同一法则。）

Avoid cold-property medicines in the cold season, cool-property medicines in the cool season, warm-property medicines in the warm season, and hot-property medicines in the hot season. This principle also applies to diet. (*Plain Conversation*)

◎ 用热远热，用寒远寒，所谓必先岁气，毋伐天和也。(《医门法律》卷一)

（用热药时要避开炎热的气候，用寒药时要避开寒冷的气候，必须先知道岁气的偏胜，不能攻伐自然冲和之气。）

Avoid hot-property medicines in the hot season and cold-property medicines in the cold season. One must be aware of the predominant qi of a season to avoid upsetting the yin-yang equilibrium of nature. (*Precepts for Physicians*) yòng rè yuǎn rè

# 用热远热

Avoid Hot-property Medicines in the Hot Season

用热远热，中医因时制宜用药思路之一，即夏月阳盛阴弱，病易化热伤阴，当慎用热药，以免助邪热燔灼之势。人体在春夏阳热之季，表现为"人气在外，皮肤缓，腠理开，血气减，汗大泄，皮淖泽"(《灵枢·刺节真邪论》)，病变多为热邪伤阴，机体阴阳失调一般呈现出阴气虚而阳气盛。因此，临床用药之时，应注意炎热季节慎用大热的药物。

The term refers to the principle of using medicines according to time in traditional Chinese medicine. In summertime, yang is predominant and yin is weak. It is easy for diseases to transform into heat and impair yin, so hot-property medicines should be used with caution to avoid the increase in pathogenic heat. In spring and summer, "Qi in the human body floats externally, skin becomes loose, muscular interstice is open, qi and blood decrease, sweat flows off massively, and skin appears moist" (*Miraculous Pivot*, "Discussion on the Five Sections in Needling and Comments on the Genuine-qi and Pathogenic Factors"). Disorders are mostly caused by pathogenic heat impairing yin, and yin-yang disharmony is manifested by yin deficiency and yang excess in the human body. Therefore, in clinical practice, medicines with great hot property should be cautiously used during the hot season.

【曾经译法】无

【现行译法】avoiding drugs of warm or hot nature in hot climate; avoiding using hot medicinals in summer; avoiding using hot-propertied (note: "hot-propertied" should be revised as "hot-property") medicines in hot weather

【推荐译法】avoid hot-property medicines in the hot season

【翻译说明】"用热远热"中第一个"热"指药性热，译为 hot-property medicines；第二个"热"指炎热之季，译为 the hot season。

"远"指"远离；避开"，译为 avoid。"用热远热"可译为
avoid hot-property medicines in the hot season。


引例 Citations:

◎ 夫子言用寒远寒，用热远热，余未知其然也，愿闻何谓远？岐伯曰：
热无犯热，寒无犯寒，从者和，逆者病，不可不敬畏而远之。(《素问·六
元正纪大论》)

（"你讲过，用寒药应该避免气候寒冷，用热药应该避免气候炎
热，我不知道这里面的道理，希望你讲一下怎样叫做避免？"岐
伯说："天热不要用热药，天寒不要用寒药。顺应这一规律则身
体平和，否则就会添病，不可不谨慎而避免它。"）

"You have stated that cold-property medicines should be avoided in the cold
season and hot-property medicines should be avoided in the hot season. I would
like to know why and what 'avoidance' means." Qibo answered: "Do not
use medicines hot in nature in hot weather, and do not use medicines cold in
nature in cold weather. To follow this principle will result in harmony, whereas
opposition will cause illness. One must be cautious enough to observe it." (*Plain
Conversation*)

◎ 用温远温，用热远热，用凉远凉，用寒远寒，无翼其胜也。故冬不用
白虎，夏不用青龙，春夏不服桂枝，秋冬不服麻黄，不失气宜。(《脾胃
论》卷上)

（用温药时要避开温暖的气候，用热药时要避开炎热的气候，用
凉药时要避开清凉的气候，用寒药时要避开寒冷的气候，不要辅
助偏胜。因此，冬天不用白虎汤，夏天不用青龙汤，春夏不服用
桂枝，秋冬不服用麻黄，不违背四时气候之宜。）

Avoid warm-property medicines in the warm season, hot-property medicines in the hot season, cool-property medicines in the cool season, and cold-property medicines in the cold season. Do not reinforce the predominant qi of a season. Therefore, *Baihu* Decoction (White Tiger Decoction) should not be used in wintertime, *Qinglong* Decoction (Bluegreen Dragon Decoction) should not be used in summertime, *guizhi* (*Ramulus Cinnamomi*, cinnamon twig) should not be used in spring or summer, and *mahuang* (*Herba Ephedrae*, ephedra) should not be used in autumn or winter. One should comply with the qi of the four seasons. (*Treatise on the Spleen and Stomach*) hánzhě rè zhī

# 寒者热之

Treat Cold with Heat

　　寒者热之，中医正治法之一，也称"治寒以热"，是指用温热方药治疗寒性病证的一种治疗原则。如过食生冷，脾胃运化功能失常，而见腹痛不止，下利稀水，伴形寒肢冷者，应以温脾健运的方法治疗。又如外感风寒，见恶寒发热、头痛、脉浮者，以辛温解表之剂治疗。寒证有表寒、里寒、虚寒、实寒之别，其相应的治法均属"寒者热之"的具体运用。

The term, also known as cold treated with heat, refers to one of the routine treatment methods in traditional Chinese medicine. It is a principle of treating cold patterns with medicines that are warm or hot in property. For instance, the therapy for warming the spleen to promote transportation and transformation is used to treat the dysfunction of the spleen and the stomach due to overeating cold foods. The disorder is characterized by persistent abdominal pain, loose stools, and cold limbs. Medicines pungent in taste and warm in property are prescribed to relieve exogenous wind-cold characterized by an aversion to cold, fever, and a floating pulse. Cold patterns encompass exterior cold, interior cold, deficiency cold, and excess cold. Their corresponding therapies all belong to the category of treating cold patterns with hot-property medicines.

【曾经译法】 treat the cold-syndrome with warm-natured drugs; heating the cold; cold-syndrome should be treated with warm-natured drugs; treating the cold-syndrome with hot-natured drugs; Coldness should be dealt with warmness; cold is treated with heat; cryopathy requiring warm prescription; treating cold syndrome with heat methods

【现行译法】 treating the cold syndrome with hot-natured drugs; cold disease should be treated by warm therapy; treat the cold with heat; Treating cold syndrome with hot-natured herbs; treating cold syndrome with hot-natured drugs; treating cold syndrome with hot methods; treating cold syndrome with warm drugs; heating the cold; treating coldness with heat; treating cold with heat; herbs hot in property prescribed for a cold syndrome; treating the cold with the hot; treat cold with heat; Cold treated with warm

【推荐译法】 treat cold with heat

【翻译说明】"寒者热之"指用温热方药治疗寒性病证，是中医治法和治疗原则。可采用 treat...with... 结构来翻译，译为 treat cold with heat。以往译法中的 cryopathy 是"寒冷病"，主要指由于冰冻造成的伤害和损伤，与中医的寒性病证有很大差异，故不建议使用。2022 年发布的《世界卫生组织中医药术语国际标准》将此术语翻译为 treat cold with heat，同时列出 cold treated with warm 为同义词组。

引例 Citations:

◎ 寒者热之，热者寒之，温者清之，清者温之。(《素问·至真要大论》)

（寒病用热药，热病用寒药，温病用凉药，凉病用温药。）

Treat cold patterns with hot-property medicines, heat patterns with cold-property medicines, warm diseases with cool-property medicines, and cool diseases with warm-property medicines. (*Plain Conversation*)

◎ 温者，温其中也，脏受寒侵，必须温剂，经云寒者热之是已。(《医学心悟》卷一)

（温者，即温暖其里。五脏受到寒邪侵袭，必须用温热的方药，《黄帝内经》说寒病用热药，就是如此。）

Warming is to warm the interior. Medicines warm and hot in property should be used when the five *zang*-organs are invaded by pathogenic cold. This is what is stated in *Huangdi's Inner Canon of Medicine*: treating cold with heat. (*Medical Understanding*) rèzhě hán zhī

# 热者寒之

## Treat Heat with Cold

热者寒之，中医正治法之一，也称"治热以寒"，是指用寒凉方药治疗热性病证的一种治疗原则。如因湿热下注大肠，见下利脓血、里急后重、身热口干、舌红苔黄、脉数等症，用苦寒燥湿，清热凉血方药治疗；又如外感风热，见发热恶风、头痛、舌红、脉数者，用辛凉解表方剂治疗。热证有表热、里热、虚热、实热之别，其治疗方法也相应地有所不同，但均属"热者寒之"的具体运用。

The term, also known as heat treated with cold, refers to one of the routine treatment methods in traditional Chinese medicine. It is a principle of treating heat patterns with medicines that are cool or cold in property. For instance, the therapy of drying dampness with bitter and cold medicines and prescriptions of clearing heat and cooling blood are used to treat dampness heat in the large intestine. The disorder is characterized by stools with pus and blood, tenesmus, increased body temperature, dry mouth, a red tongue with yellow coating, and a rapid pulse. Formulas that release the exterior with pungent cool medicines are used to relieve externally contracted wind heat manifested as fever, an aversion to wind, headache, a red tongue, and a rapid pulse. Heat patterns encompass exterior heat, interior heat, deficiency heat, and excess heat. Their corresponding therapies, though varying accordingly, all belong to the category of treating heat patterns with cold-property medicines.

【曾经译法】 treat the heat-syndrome with cold-natured drugs; cooling the heat; heat-syndrome should be treated with cold-natured drugs; heat syndrome being treated with drugs of cold or cool nature; Heat syndromes should be treated with cooling therapy; heat is treated with cold; expelling heat with cold herbs; heat syndrome treated with drugs of cold or cool nature; treating heat syndrome with cold methods

【现行译法】treating heat syndrome with drugs cool or cold in nature; treating heat syndrome with cold therapy; treat the heat with cold; Heat is treated with cold; Heat Syndrome Treated with Cold or Cool Drugs; heat syndrome being treated with drugs of cold or cool nature; treating heat syndrome with cold methods; treating heat syndrome with cold-natured drugs; cooling the heat; treating hotness with coldness; treating heat with cold; herbs cold in property prescribed for a heat syndrome; treating heat syndrome with the cold; treat heat with cold; Heat treated with cold

【推荐译法】treat heat with cold

【翻译说明】"热者寒之"指用寒凉方药治疗热性病证，是中医治法和治疗原则。可采用 treat...with... 结构来翻译，译为 treat heat with cold。2022 年发布的《世界卫生组织中医药术语国际标准》将此术语翻译为 treat heat with cold，同时列出 heat treated with cold 为同义词组。

引例 Citations:

◎ 凡治诸胜复，太阳气寒，则寒者热之；少阴少阳气热，则热者寒之。
（《黄帝内经素问注证发微》卷九）

（凡是治疗各种胜气、报复之气所致的病证，太阳为寒气，故寒病用热药；少阴、少阳为热气，故热病用寒药。）

Any disorder caused by prevailing qi or retaliating qi is ascribed to cold in *taiyang* meridian, and heat in *shaoyin* and *shaoyang* meridians. The former should follow the principle of treating cold with heat, whereas the latter should follow the principle of treating heat with cold. (*An Elaboration of "Plain Conversation" in Huangdi's Inner Canon of Medicine*)

◎ 凡治火者，实热之火，可以寒胜，可以水折，所谓热者寒之也。(《景
岳全书·传忠录》)

（凡是治疗火证者，实热火邪，可以用寒药清泻，可以用水制约，
这就是所说的热病用寒药治疗。）

To cure fire patterns characterized by excess heat and pathogenic fire, cold-property medicines are used to purge or water is used to restrain. This is called treating heat with cold. (*Complete Works of Jingyue*) jiānzhě bìngxíng

# 间者并行

## Treat Both Tip and Root in a Mild Case

间者并行，中医标本论治方法与原则，语出《素问·标本病传论》，指病情轻浅者宜标本兼治。张介宾《类经·论治类》说："间者言病之浅……病浅者可以兼治，故曰并行。"因为在临床上，凡标本病势均等，则单治标病或单治本病，往往达不到治愈疾病的效果，只有标本兼治，收效才会好。如阴血亏虚之人外感风寒之邪，则治宜加减葳蕤汤之类，扶正祛邪，标本同治。当然，在标本同治时，尚应分清主次，而有所侧重，或治本顾标，或治标顾本。

The term refers to one of the treatment methods and principles based on differentiation between *biao* (tip, manifestation or symptom) and *ben* (root or root cause). Derived from *Plain Conversation* ("Discussion on the Transmission of Tip and Root"), it means treating manifestations and root cause simultaneously in a mild case. "*Jian* (间) means a mild disease... For a mild case, treat both tip and root simultaneously," stated Zhang Jiebin in the "On Treatment" of his *Classified Classics*. Clinical practice proves that good results could be obtained if both tip and root are treated simultaneously when the two result in a draw. Treating either tip or root only cannot achieve a cure on such occasions. For instance, in the case of yin-blood deficiency affected by pathogenic wind cold, *Jiajian Weirui* Decoction (Solomon's Seal Variant Decoction) should be prescribed to reinforce healthy qi and eliminate pathogenic factors simultaneously, that is, to treat both the tip and the root. Nevertheless, when treating both the tip and the root, one should distinguish the primary cause from the secondary one: focus on the root or the tip according to the reality.

【曾经译法】 a mild case should be dealt with the treatment aiming at both the primary and secondary symptoms; simultaneous application of principal and subordinate treatments

【现行译法】 treating main and accompanying symptoms of a mild disease simultaneously; chronic case necessary to treat both primary and secondary symptoms; treating root and accompanying symptoms simultaneously for mild case; if the illness is mild, treat the root and tip

【推荐译法】 treat both tip and root in a mild case

【翻译说明】 "间者并行"指病情轻浅者宜标本兼治。"病情轻浅者"不能译为 chronic case（慢性病），译为 mild case（轻症）较妥。中医语境中，"标"常被译为 tip/manifestation/symptom，"本"常用 root/root cause 表示。单词 tip（尖端；树梢）和 root（根）能够比较形象地体现主次关系，因此，建议将"间者并行"译为 treat both tip and root in a mild case。


引例 Citations:


◎ 谨察间甚，以意调之，间者并行，甚者独行。（《素问·标本病传论》）

（要谨慎地观察病情的轻重，根据具体病情用心调治，病轻的可以标本兼治，病重的就要根据具体病情，或治标或治本。）

One should carefully investigate whether the disease is mild or severe and treat the disease with full attention. Treat both tip and root in a mild case; treat either tip or root in a severe case according to the patient's condition. (*Plain Conversation*)

◎ 间者并行，甚者独行。盖并者并也，传其所间而病势并行也；独者特也，特传其所胜也。（《黄帝内经素问注证发微》卷二）

（病轻的可以标本兼治，病重的就要根据具体病情，或治标或治本。大概并者，兼并，病传其子而病势并行；独者，单一，单传其五行所胜之脏。）

Treat both tip and root in a mild case, and treat either tip or root in a severe one according to the patient's condition. Generally, a severe case results from the mother-organ disease affecting the child-organ and both are acute, whereas a mild case involves a single organ—the one being overcome among the five elements. (*An Elaboration of "Plain Conversation"* in *Huangdi's Inner Canon of Medicine*) shènzhě dúxíng

# 甚者独行

Treat Either Tip or Root in a Severe Case

甚者独行，中医标本论治方法与原则，语出《素问·标本病传论》，指病情深重者宜单治标或单治本。张介宾《类经·论治类》说："甚者言病之重也……病甚者难容杂乱，故曰独行。"在临床上，如病情较重的，可视其标或本的某一方病势较急而又易于取效者，则先专力治之，本急标缓则治本，标急本缓则治标。

The term refers to one of the treatment methods and principles based on differentiation between *biao* (tip, manifestation or symptom) and *ben* (root or root cause). Derived from *Plain Conversation* ("Discussion on the Transmission of Tip and Root"), it means treating either tip or root in a severe case. "*Shen* (甚) means severity… It means the disease is complex and complicated; therefore, it is better to treat either tip or root," stated Zhang Jiebin in the "On Treatment" of his *Classified Classics*. For severe cases, clinical treatment should focus on the aspect that is acute and easy to achieve a cure. Treat the root first if it is in an acute condition while the tip is not, and treat the tip first if it is in an acute condition while the root is not.

【曾经译法】a severe case should be treated with potent drugs of specific action; focal treatment for serious disease

【现行译法】treating severe cases by a single method; focal treatment of serious disease; severe case treated with potent drugs of specific action; treating a serious case with formulas of strong and specific action; treating severe case with single focal method; the serious case being treated by only specific therapy; if the illness is serious, treat the root or tip

【推荐译法】treat either tip or root in a severe case

【翻译说明】"甚者独行"指患者病情严重时，宜单独治标或单独治本。中医语境中，"标"常被译为 tip/manifestation/symptom，"本"常用 root/root cause 表示。单词 tip（尖端；树梢）和 root（根）能够比较形象地体现主次关系，因此，建议将"甚者独行"译为 treat either tip or root in a severe case。

引例 Citations:

◎ 间者并行，甚者独行，此标本之大法也。（《素问直解·标本病传论》）

（病轻的可以标本兼治，病重的就要根据具体病情，或治本或治标，这是标本论治的大法。）

Treat both tip and root in a mild case, and treat either tip or root in a severe one according to the patient's condition. This is the guideline for treatment based on differentiation between tip and root. (*Direct Interpretation of "Plain Conversation"*)

◎ 间者并行，谓病势轻者，标本可以兼治；甚者独行，谓病势甚者，或宜治本，或宜治标，一意专行，勿或瞻狗也。（《素问释义·标本病传论》）

（间者并行，是说病势轻者，标本可以兼治；甚者独行，是说病势严重者，或应治本，或应治标，专心一意，不能以自己的喜好而违反该治则。）

Treat both tip and root in a mild case, that is, to address both symptoms and root cause simultaneously for the patient with a mild illness. Treat either tip or root in a severe case according to the patient's condition. Basically, one should have undivided attention and should not violate these principles. (*Interpretation of "Plain Conversation"*) wēizhě nì zhī

# 微者逆之

Treat a Mild Disease by Opposing

微者逆之，中医治法之一，语出《素问·至真要大论》，指对于病变较轻，病情单纯，疾病表象与本质相一致的病证，采用药物的性质、作用趋向违逆疾病表象而治的方法，即逆治法，也称为"正治法"。如寒证用热药，热证用寒药等。

The term, derived from *Plain Conversation* ("Significant Discussions on the Most Important and Abstruse Theory"), refers to one of the routine treatment methods in traditional Chinese medicine. It means using medicines whose property and action are opposite to the exhibited manifestations to address mild and non-complicated cases, in which their symptoms and natures are consistent. For example, treat cold patterns with medicines hot in nature and treat heat patterns with medicines cold in nature.

【曾经译法】 mild illness dealt with by routine treatment; opposing the mild; mild case should be treated with the routine treatment; Mild illness should be treated by routine treatment; treating mild cases with routine principle; mild conditions are treated by counteraction; routine therapy for mild case; mild conditions are treated directly

【现行译法】 treating mild illness by routine treatment; treating mild syndrome with contrary therapy/treating mild cases with routine principle; treat mild and simple cases with drugs opposite in nature to the disease; opposing the mild; treating mild syndrome with counteraction; mild disease being routinely treated; mild disease being treated routinely; treat mild and simple cases by counteracting principle

【推荐译法】treat a mild disease by opposing

【翻译说明】正治法或逆治法包括寒者热之、热者寒之、虚者补之、实者泄之等多种情况，用表示"正治法"的 routine treatment/principle 或 being treated routinely 来翻译"逆之"，含义过于宽泛；counteraction 或 counteracting 常表示"对抗；抵消；中和"，不能体现"逆之"的确切内涵。为照顾术语的简洁性和类似术语结构的一致性，建议将"微者逆之"翻译为 treat a mild disease by opposing。


引例 Citations:


◎ 夫病之微小者，犹人火也，遇草而焫，得木而燔，可以湿伏，可以水灭，故逆其性气以折之攻之。(《重广补注黄帝内经素问》卷二十二)

（疾病轻微者，犹如人为过失造成的火灾，遇到草就燃，遇树木就焚，可用湿制伏，可用水灭火。因此，逆病性以损折、攻伐它。）

A mild case is like a fire disaster caused by human error. Grasses and trees can be burnt in a fire. But dampness and water can quench the fire. Hence, the disease can be treated with medicines opposite in nature for a counterattack. (*Huangdi's Inner Canon of Medicine: Broadly Corrected and Re-annotated*)

◎ 盖微者逆之，逆者正治，此理之正也；甚者从之，从者反治，此理之权也。(《圣济总录》卷四)

（轻者逆着病情来治疗，逆病情来治疗就是正治，这是医理的常规；重者顺着病情来治疗，顺着病情来治疗就是反治，这是医理的权变。）

Mild cases are treated by opposing. Applying treatment opposite to the state of a disease is routine treatment, which is the normal or standard medical practice. Severe cases are treated by following. Treating diseases by following their manifestations is paradoxical treatment, which is the adapted form of medical practice. (*Comprehensive Records of Sacred Benevolence*) shènzhě cóng zhī

# 甚者从之

Treat a Severe Disease by Following

甚者从之，中医治法之一，语出《素问·至真要大论》，指对于病变较重、病情复杂、疾病表象与本质不完全一致的病证，采用药物的性质、作用趋向顺从疾病表象而治的方法，即从治法，也称为"反治法"。如寒病表现出热象，热病表现出寒象，虚证表现出闭塞之象，积滞、瘀阻者表现出泻利之象等，顺从疾病表象而治，所谓"热因热用，寒因寒用，塞因塞用，通因通用"。

The term, derived from *Plain Conversation* ("Significant Discussions on the Most Important and Abstruse Theory"), refers to one of the paradoxical treatment methods in traditional Chinese medicine. It means using medicines whose property and action are in accordance with the exhibited manifestations to address the cases that are severe and complicated and whose symptoms and natures are not completely consistent. For example, heat symptoms are exhibited in cold patterns, cold symptoms in heat patterns, blockage symptoms in deficiency patterns, and diarrhea in stagnation and stasis patterns. In such conditions, it is advised to treat diseases by following the manifestations of the diseases, for example, to treat heat with heat, treat cold with cold, treat the blocked by blocking, and treat the flowing by promoting flow.

【曾经译法】 serious illness should be dealt with by the treatment opposite to the routine; following the severe (note: a mistranslation); the serious case should be treated contrary to the routine treatment; Severe cases with pseudo-symptoms should be treated with drugs similar in nature to the pseudo-symptoms; treating severe cases according to the nature of the existing symptoms; severe conditions are treated by coaction; in severe cases follow the symptoms

【现行译法】treating severe cases with pseudo-symptoms by using drugs similar in nature to the pseudo-symptoms; treat complicated cases with drugs similar in nature to the pseudo-symptoms; severe case with pseudo-symptoms having to be treated with drugs similar in nature to pseudo-symptoms; following the severe (note: a mistranslation); treating severe case in compliance with pseudosymptom; treating a severe case with herbs, the nature of which is in compliance with pseudosymptoms; serious case being treated contrarily; treat complicated cases by co-acting principle

【推荐译法】treat a severe disease by following

【翻译说明】从治法或反治法包括热因热用、寒因寒用、塞因塞用、通因通用等多种情况，用 opposite to the routine, contrary to the routine treatment 或 being treated contrarily 等不能直接体现"从之"的内涵。为照顾术语的简洁性和类似术语结构的一致性，建议将"甚者从之"翻译为 treat a severe disease by following。

引例 Citations:

◎ 方热之微，而寒治之，治之不已，则热格寒而益加，故因寒而用热，此之谓从之以导其甚，《至真要大论》曰：微者逆之，甚者从之，此之谓也。（《圣济经》卷十）

（正当热势轻时，用寒药治疗它，治疗而不愈，就会阳热格拒阴寒而病情加重，因此由于寒而用热药，这就是顺从它以引导其热。《至真要大论》说：轻者逆着病情来治疗，重者顺着病情来治疗，说的就是这种情况。）

When heat is mild, use cold medicines to relieve it. If not cured, the condition will deteriorate due to yang heat rejecting yin cold. Therefore, using medicines hot in property to relieve pseudo-cold symptoms is in accordance with the disease nature to release heat. According to *Plain Conversation* ("Significant Discussions on the Most Important and Abstruse Theory"), "Treat a mild disease by opposing and a severe one by following. This is exactly the case." (*Classic of Sacred Benevolence*)

◎ 其色青而带白，是为贼邪难治，故多死，法曰甚者从之，谓反治也。
(《医学正传》卷一)

> （面色青而带有白色，这是贼邪，病情难治，因此预后不良。治
> 法言病情重者顺着病情来治疗，称为"反治"。）

Bluish complexion with whitish color indicates an invasion of pathogenic factors. It is difficult to achieve a cure and the prognosis is poor. In terms of the method, treating a severe disease by following its pseudo-symptoms is called "paradoxical treatment." (*Orthodoxy of Medicine*) kèzhě chú zhī

# 客者除之

Treat What Invades by Eliminating

客者除之，中医治法之一，是指针对感受外邪所导致的病证，运用祛除邪气的方法治疗。客，指外来邪气，包括风、寒、暑、湿、燥、火六淫、疫疬之邪，以及饮食积滞等。除，有祛除、驱逐之义。如疏风、散寒、清暑、祛湿、泻火、消导等法，均属客者除之的范畴。外邪客于表，则治以解表发汗法；病邪客于里，则治以攻里通下法等。

The term refers to one of the treatment methods in traditional Chinese medicine. It means treating patterns caused by exogenous pathogens by eliminating them. Exogenous pathogens encompass six pathogenic factors (wind, cold, summer heat, dampness, dryness, and fire), epidemic pestilence, and food stagnation. Eliminating methods include removing wind, dissipating cold, clearing summer heat, draining dampness, purging fire, and promoting digestion. When exogenous pathogenic factors invade the exterior, treatment should focus on releasing the exterior and promoting sweating; when they invade the interior, treatment should focus on purging the interior and promoting bowel movements.

【曾经译法】 the exogenous evils attacking the body should be eliminated; eliminating external pathogens; exogenous evils attacking the body should be eliminated; what intrudes is eliminated; expelling exogenous pathogens; eliminate what intrudes; expelling exogenous pathogens

【现行译法】 treating excess syndrome by eliminating pathogenic factors; remove what is intruding; To eliminate exopathogens; eliminating external pathogens; exogenous pathogen should be expelled; eliminating invaded pathogenic factors; the invaded being eliminated

【推荐译法】treat what invades by eliminating

【翻译说明】"客者"既包括外来邪气，也包括食积等内生之邪，因此不能将"客者"只理解为外邪，译为 exogenous evils/pathogens，external pathogens 或 exopathogens，建议译为 what invades，比 the invaded pathogenic factors 更简洁。为照顾术语的简洁性和类似术语结构的一致性，建议将"客者除之"译为 treat what invades by eliminating。

引例 Citations:

◎ 以黄连、黄芩、黄柏、知母、连翘、生地黄、龙胆草，诸去除热邪为使，为客者除之也。(《原机启微》卷下)

（用黄连、黄芩、黄柏、知母、连翘、生地黄、龙胆草，各种去除热邪药物为使者，是邪气留于体内就驱逐它。）

Heat-removing medicines such as *Huanglian* (*Rhizoma Coptidis*, coptis rhizome), *Huangqin* (*Radix Scutellariae*, scutellaria root), *Huangbo* (*Cortex Phellodendri Chinensis*, amur cork-tree bark), *Zhimu* (*Rhizoma Anemarrhenae*, common anemarrhena rhizome), *Lianqiao* (*Fructus Forsythiae*, weeping forsythia capsule), *Sheng Dihuang* (*Radix Rehmanniae*, raw rehmannia), and *Longdancao* (*Radix et Rhizoma Gentianae*, Chinese gentian) are used as guides to remove heat pathogens. This is the method of treating what invades by eliminating. (*Revealing the Mystery of the Origin of Eye Diseases*)

◎ 骨皮饮治阳邪之陷于肝脏也，客者除之，勿纵寇以遗患也。(《名医方论》卷二)

（骨皮饮治疗阳邪内陷于肝，邪气留于体内就驱逐它，不要放任贼寇而遗留后患。）

*Gu Pi* Drink (Chinese Wolfberry Bark Drink) is used to treat yang pathogen entering the liver. This invaded pathogen should be eliminated to fend off potential risks. (*Discussion on Famous Physicians' Formulas*) láozhě wēn zhī

# 劳者温之

Treat Consumptive Diseases by Mild Tonification

劳者温之，中医治法之一，又称"损者温之"，是指针对各种慢性消耗性疾病，正气亏虚损伤，采用甘温滋补的药物进行温养。正气虚劳损伤的病证，理应包括一切正气不足所致的疾病，但这里提出用温性药物补养，所以主要是针对气虚、阳虚、血虚三类虚损劳伤病证而设，若气虚者用甘温益气之法，阳虚者用温补阳气之法，血虚者也当用甘温之药治疗。如虚劳内伤，中气不足所致的身热汗出，渴喜热饮，少气懒言，脉象虚大等，用补中益气汤甘温除热法治疗等。

The term, also known as "consumptive diseases treated with warm-property tonics," refers to one of the treatment methods in traditional Chinese medicine. It means using tonics that are sweet in taste and warm in property to treat various chronic consumptive conditions including deficiency and impairment of healthy qi. Diseases resulting from deficiency and impairment of healthy qi should have encompassed all kinds of disorders due to insufficiency of healthy qi, but the term emphasizes tonification with warm-property medicines. Therefore, consumptive diseases here are limited to the disorders caused by qi deficiency, yang deficiency, and blood deficiency. For qi deficiency, reinforce qi with sweet, warm medicines; for yang deficiency, warm and replenish qi; for blood deficiency, use sweet, warm medicines. When a patient has fever, sweating, thirst and a desire for hot drinks, shallow breathing with little desire to talk, and a deficient, large pulse caused by consumptive diseases resulting in insufficiency of spleen-stomach qi, *Buzhong Yiqi* Decoction (Decoction for Tonifying Middle *Jiao* and Boosting Qi) is prescribed, which is an example of eliminating heat with sweet, warm medicines.

【曾经译法】asthenic diseases should be invigorated with drugs of warm nature; warming the consumptive; a case of general debility should be invigorated with warm-natured drugs; warming the

125

over-exhausted; Consumptive syndrome should be treated with warm herbs; taxation (note: taxing, an adjective, means "physically or mentally demanding") is treated by warming; Taxation (note: taxing, an adjective, means "physically or mentally demanding") is treated with warm drugs (drugs in warm nature)

【现行译法】 warming the over-exhausted; treatment of consumptive disease with herbs; give warming tonics to the debilitated; General debility treated with warm-natured drugs; Warming Consumption; warming the consumptive; treating overstrain with warming; debilitated patients treated with herbs warm in property; warming therapy for overstrain diseases

【推荐译法】 treat consumptive diseases by mild tonification

【翻译说明】 "劳者温之"，又称"损者温之"，指采用甘温滋补的药物治疗各种慢性消耗性疾病。后世一般不区分"劳者"和"损者"，可译为 consumptive diseases，而不是 asthenic diseases（虚性疾病）、general debility（全身虚弱）、the over-exhausted（疲劳过度者）、taxation（耗费）或 overstrain（过度紧张）。"温之"意思是"温和补养它"，译为 treat...by mild tonification，而不只是 warm-natured drugs（温性药），因为并不是所有温性药都有补益作用。因此，建议将"劳者温之"译为 treat consumptive diseases by mild tonification。


引例 Citations:


◎《内经》曰劳者温之，损者温之，盖温能除大热，大忌苦寒之药泻胃土耳，今立补中益气汤。(《内外伤辨》卷中)

（《黄帝内经》说：病属劳倦所致的就温养它，病属虚损的就温补它。温药能解除大热，最忌用苦寒药物以攻泻脾胃，现创立补中益气汤。)

*Huangdi's Inner Canon of Medicine* states: "Treat overstrain syndrome with mild tonifying medicines; treat deficiency and consumption with warm-property tonics." Warm-property medicines can remove intense heat. Bitter, cold medicines for purging the spleen and the stomach should be prohibited from use. Thus, *Buzhong Yiqi* Deoction (Decoction for Tonifying Middle *Jiao* and Boosting Qi) is formulated. (*Differentiation of Damage from Internal and External Causes*)

◎ 经曰劳者温之，温谓温存而养之，今之医者，以温为温之药，差之久矣。(《儒门事亲》卷三)

（《黄帝内经》说病属劳倦所致的就温养它，温是说温和补养，现在的医生，认为温为温性的药物，相差久远了。)

*Huangdi's Inner Canon of Medicine* states: "Treat consumptive diseases by mild tonification." Physicians presently mistake "mildness" for "warm-property medicines." It is far from the truth. (*Confucians' Duties to Their Parents*) jiézhě sàn zhī

# 结者散之

Treat Accumulations by Dissipating

　　结者散之，中医治法之一，是指针对气、血、痰、火等郁结的病证，运用疏散或消散的方药治疗。如气滞者治以行气导滞法；血瘀者治以活血化瘀法；痰热互结心下，胸脘痞满，按之则痛，用宽胸散结法治疗等。类似治法如"坚者削之"，指体内有坚硬积块，如癥瘕、积聚之类，运用活血化瘀、软坚散结等削伐方药治疗。

The term refers to one of the treatment methods in traditional Chinese medicine. It means using medicines that disperse or dissipate to relieve qi stagnation, blood stasis, and accumulations of phlegm and fire. For qi stagnation, qi is promoted to remove stagnation; for blood stasis, blood circulation is promoted to remove stasis. For phlegm-fire accumulation below the heart characterized by chest and gastric stuffiness and tenderness upon pressing, the method of improving qi circulation and dissipating accumulation is used. Similar treatment methods include "treating hardness by reducing" which refers to the use of medicines that promote qi circulation to remove stasis and soften hardness to dissipate accumulations in the body such as abdominal masses.

【曾经译法】 disease resulting from accumulation of evil should be treated with dispersing therapy; disease caused by accumulation of evils should be treated with therapy of dispersion; binding is treated by dissipation; stagnation requiring dispersion

【现行译法】 treating lumps with repellents; resolve what is bound together; Treating clumping by dispersing; Dispersing Nodules and Masses; treating pathogenic accumulation with dissipation; enlarged nodes requiring dissipation; binding being dissipated; dissipate what are bound together

【推荐译法】 treat accumulations by dissipating

【翻译说明】"结者"包括气、血、痰、火等郁结的病证，译为 accumulations，内涵比较宽泛，可以涵盖 stagnation（瘀滞）、nodules and masses（结节和肿块）和 enlarged nodes（淋巴结肿大）等多种病症。"散"的译文目前有 disperse/dispersion 和 dissipate/dissipation 两种：disperse 意思是分散、驱散，东西被散开了但还存在；dissipate 意思是消散而不存在，更符合"散结"的意思。


引例 Citations:


◎ 大热药中兼用结者散之，乃神药也。（《医学启源》序）

（大热的药物中，兼用疏散气血郁结的药物，是神奇的药物。）


Among the medicines with great hot property, those that can also remove qi stagnation and blood stasis are the miracle cures. (*The Origin of Medicine*)


◎ 以柴胡、防风、羌活、细辛、藁本，诸升阳化滞为臣，为结者散之也。（《原机启微》卷下）

（用柴胡、防风、羌活、细辛、藁本，各种升阳化滞药为臣药，就是病属气血郁结而加以疏散治疗的方法。）


Herbs such as *chaihu* (*Radix Bupleuri*, Chinese thorowax root), *fangfeng* (*Radix Saposhnokoviae*, divaricate saposhnikovia root), *qianghuo* (*Rhizomaseu Radix Notopterygii*, notopterygium rhizome or root), *xixin* (*Herba Asari*, manchurian wild ginger), and *gaoben* (*Rhizoma Ligustici*, Chinese lovage) are used as minister medicines to promote yang qi and resolve stagnations. This is the method of treating accumulations by dissipating. (*Revealing the Mystery of the Origin of Eye Diseases*) liúzhě gōng zhī

# 留者攻之

Treat Retention by Purging

留者攻之，中医治法之一，是指针对饮食停滞、蓄水、血瘀经闭等瘀滞病证，运用攻逐泻下的方药治疗。留，指停留不去；攻，即攻逐之义。如悬饮，胁下有水气，症见咳嗽，胸胁引痛，心下痞硬，干呕短气，头痛目眩，或胸背掣痛不得息及水肿腹胀，属实证者，用攻逐水饮法治疗。

The term refers to one of the treatment methods in traditional Chinese medicine. It means using purgative medicines to treat food accumulation, water retention, and amenorrhea due to blood stasis. Retention means remaining in the body; purging means removing. Pleural fluid retention with fluid retained in hypochondriac regions, for example, is characterized by cough accompanied by chest and hypochondriac pain, distention and tightness below the heart, retching, shortness of breath, headache, and dizziness, or by breathing difficulty due to referred pain in the chest and back as well as edema and abdominal distention. It is an excess pattern and purgative method should be used.

【曾经译法】 the endogenous evil factors remained in the body should be driven out; expelling the stagnant; disease with retention of evil in the body should be treated by elimination; lodging is treated by attack; retention requiring purgation

【现行译法】 removing retained pathogenic factors from the body; treatment of retention with purgation; attack what is lingering; expelling the stagnant; treating retention with purgation; launching attack against retained pathogenic factors; the lodged being treated by attacking

【推荐译法】 treat retention by purging

【翻译说明】 "留"指停留不去，译为 retention 较妥。译词 linger 常表示"徘徊；逗留；苟延残喘"；stagnant 常表示"停滞的；无发

展变化的"。"攻"指攻逐。为照顾术语的简洁性和类似术语
结构的一致性，建议将"留者攻之"译为 treat retention by
purging。

引例 Citations:

◎ 况乎留饮下无补法，气方隔塞，补则转增，岂知《内经》所谓留者攻之，
何后人不师古之甚也。（《儒门事亲》卷三）

（何况治疗留饮在用下法时并无同用补法之理。因为气正阻隔闭
塞之下，补益就会反而加重病情。这哪里是懂得了《黄帝内经》
所说的"留者攻之"之义呢！为什么后人这么不遵从古人的教
诲呢！）

Moreover, there is no reason to use purgative method in combination with
tonifying method to treat prolonged fluid retention because tonification will
aggravate the disease when qi is obstructed. How can they say they understand
the implication of "treating retention by purging" in *Huangdi's Inner Canon
of Medicine*? Why is it so serious that later generations would not follow the
ancients? (*Confucians' Duties to Their Parents*)

◎ 内因积食生冷而成，留者攻之，故用阿魏棱术以去积。（《瘴疟指南》
卷下）

（由于内伤积食生冷而发病，病邪滞留的就加以攻逐，因此，用
阿魏、三棱、莪术以消除积滞。）

Retention arises from eating raw and cold food, and internal dysfunction occurs.
Retention is treated by purging. Therefore, use *awei* (*Ferulae Resina*, Chinese
asafoetida sinkiang ferula), *sanleng* (*Rhizoma Sparganii*, common burreed
tuber), and *e'zhu* (*Rhizoma Curcumae*, zedoary rhizome) to eliminate stagnation.
(*Guidelines for Miasmic Malaria*)

zàozhě rú zhī

# 燥者濡之

Treat Dryness by Moistening

    燥者濡之，即燥者润之，中医治法之一，是指针对体内津液不足所致的干燥病证，运用具有润燥生津作用的方药治疗。燥，指津液缺乏的燥证；润，即滋润之义。如阴虚肺燥的干咳，用滋阴润肺止咳法；肠燥便秘宜用润肠通便法等。

The term refers to one of the treatment methods in traditional Chinese medicine. It means using medicines that moisten dryness and generate fluids to treat dryness caused by insufficient body fluids. Dryness refers to dryness patterns due to fluid deficiency; moistening means nourishing. If one has a dry cough due to yin deficiency and lung dryness, the method of nourishing yin and moistening the lung can be used to relieve cough. For constipation caused by intestinal dryness, the method of moistening intestines and promoting bowel movements is used to relieve constipation.

【曾经译法】 treat the dryness-syndrome by therapy of moisturizing; moistening the dry; dryness-syndrome should be treated with moisturizing therapy; Dryness syndrome is treated with moistening therapy; dryness is treated by moistening; dryness requiring moistening

【现行译法】 treating dryness syndrome by moistening therapy; dryness should be treated by moistening therapy; moisten what is dried; Dryness syndrome treated by moistening therapy; Moistening Dryness; moistening the dry; treating dryness with moistening; moistening therapy for a dryness syndrome; dry syndrome being treated with moistening therapy; moisten what is dry

【推荐译法】 treat dryness by moistening

【翻译说明】 "燥"指津液缺乏的燥证，可省译为 dryness；"润"指滋润，可译为 moisten（使……湿润），比 moisture（增加水分；变潮湿）更贴近原意。为照顾术语的简洁性和类似术语结构的一致性，建议将"燥者濡之"译为 treat dryness by moistening。

引例 Citations:

◎ 燥者濡之，生地、熟地皆濡物也。（《医方考绳愆》卷二）

（病属枯燥的就加以滋润，生地、熟地都是滋润之物。）

Treat dryness by moistening. Both *shengdi* (*Radix Rehmanniae*, rehmannia root) and *shudi* (*Radix Rehmanniae Praeparata*, prepared rehmannia root) are medicines for moistening. (*Correcting Errors in the Investigations of Medical Formulas*)

◎ 滋阴润肠丸，治大肠秘结，血少肠枯，久不大便……经曰燥者濡之，此之谓也。（《胞与堂丸散谱》）

（滋阴润肠丸，治疗大肠干涩难通，血少肠道干枯，日久不大便……《黄帝内经》说"燥者濡之"，指的就是这种情况。）

*Ziyin Runchang* Pill (Pill for Nourishing Yin and Moistening Intestines) treats dryness in the large intestine due to blood insufficiency and the resultant constipation for days... This is what is stated in *Huangdi's Inner Canon of Medicine*: "Treat dryness by moistening." (*Pills and Powders for All Humanity: A Pharmacopoeia*) jízhě huǎn zhī

# 急者缓之

Treat Cramps and Rigidity by Relaxing; Relieve Acute
Symptoms

急者缓之，中医治法之一，是指针对拘急强直一类病症，运用舒展柔养、缓急解痉法治疗。急者，指拘急强直之证；缓，即缓和、缓解之义。如肝肾阴虚，阴不潜阳所致肝风内动的抽搐，用滋补肝肾、息风潜阳法治疗。又如寒邪侵袭所致的筋脉拘急，用温经散寒法治疗。由于词的多义性，该术语也可指病势急剧时采取的缓解方法。

The term refers to a treatment method in traditional Chinese medicine. It means relieving disorders such as cramps, rigidity, and tetany by relaxing and easing. *Jizhe* (急者) refers to the pattern characterized by cramps and rigidity; *huan* (缓, relaxing) means easing and mitigation. For example, the method of nourishing the liver and the kidney to stop wind and submerge yang is used to relieve convulsions caused by internal stirring of liver wind that results from liver-kidney yin deficiency and yin failing to submerge yang. The method of warming meridians and dissipating cold is used to treat muscle cramps due to the invasion of cold pathogen. Because of the polysemy of *ji* (急), the term may also mean relieving acute symptoms.

【曾经译法】 the condition with spasms should be relaxed; slowing the hurried; the spasmodic disease should be relaxed; tension is treated by relaxation; relaxing spasmodic disease

【现行译法】 tension can be relieved by relaxation; relieve what goes into spasm; Applying Relaxing Method for Acute Case; slowing the hurried; treating spasm with relaxation; relieving spasm with relaxation; tension being relieved by relaxation

【推荐译法】 1) treat cramps and rigidity by relaxing; 2) relieve acute symptoms

【翻译说明】作为一种中医治法，"急者缓之"指运用舒展柔养、缓急解痉法治疗拘急强直一类的病症。以往译法中的 spasm 表示"痉挛"；spasmodic disease 表示"痉挛性疾病；突发性疾病"；tension 常表示"紧张；拉伸"。"拘急强直"译为 cramps and rigidity 较妥。为照顾术语的简洁性和类似术语结构的一致性，"急者缓之"可译为 treat cramps and rigidity by relaxing；当"急者缓之"表示"对于病势急剧的缓解方法"时，可译为 relieve acute symptoms。


引例 Citations:


◎ 炙甘草之甘温……若脾胃急痛，腹中急缩者宜多用之，经云急者缓之。（《丹溪心法附余》卷三）

（炙甘草味甘性温……假如脾胃拘急疼痛，腹中拘急挛缩者，多用炙甘草，《黄帝内经》说病属拘急的予以缓解拘挛。）

*Zhi gancao* (*Radix et Rhizoma Glycyrrhizae Praeparata cum Melle*, prepared licorice root) is sweet in taste and warm in property… It is often used to treat acute pain in the spleen and stomach and abdominal cramps. *Huangdi's Inner Canon of Medicine* states: "Treat cramps and rigidity by relaxing." (*Appendices to Danxi's Experiential Therapy*)

◎ 东垣治例，腹痛以芍药为君，恶寒而痛加桂、甘草，缓带脉之急缩，用以为臣，经曰急者缓之。（《赤水玄珠·医案》卷一）

（李东垣治疗案例，腹痛用芍药为君药，恶寒而疼痛，加桂枝、甘草，缓解带脉的拘挛，用作臣药，《黄帝内经》说病属拘急的予以缓解拘挛。）

Li Dongyuan treated abdominal pain with *shaoyao* (*Radix Paeoniae Alba seu Rubra*, peony root) as monarch medicine, and added *guizhi* (*Ramulus Cinnamomi*, cinnamon twig) and *gancao* (*Radix et Rhizoma Glycyrrhizae*, licorice root) as minister medicines to ease cramps and rigidity of the belt vessel if the patient has pain with an aversion to cold. *Huangdi's Inner Canon of Medicine* states: "Treat cramps and rigidity by relaxing." (*Chishui and Xuanzhu: The Dao of Traditional Chinese Medicine*) sànzhě shōu zhī

# 散者收之

Treat Dissipation by Astringing

散者收之，中医治法之一，是指针对精气耗散，失于固摄和约束的病证，运用具有收敛固涩作用的方药治疗。散，即精气耗散，泛指不固不收的病证；收，指收敛固涩的作用。如心血亏虚，心气不固，以致心悸易惊，治当养血安神，以收摄心气。肾气不固的遗精滑泄，日久不愈，可用固肾涩精的方药治疗，肾气固则遗精滑泄自止。

The term refers to one of the treatment methods in traditional Chinese medicine. It means using astringent medicines to treat the pattern characterized by dissipation of essential qi and dysfunction in security and astringency. Dissipation means consumption of essential qi, referring to the patterns involving all kinds of insecurity and non-astringency. Astringing refers to having securing and astringent function. If one has heart-blood deficiency and heart-qi insecurity resulting in palpitations and susceptibility to fright, one should be treated by nourishing blood and calming the mind to secure heart qi. If one has kidney qi insecurity resulting in prolonged nocturnal emissions and spermatorrhoea, one can be treated with medicines that reinforce the kidney and astringe the essence. If kidney qi is secured, nocturnal emissions and spermatorrhoea will be prevented.

【曾经译法】 syndrome in which essence of life fails to retain in the body should be treated with astringents; gathering the dispersed; energy-wasting syndrome should be treated with astringent therapy; dissipation is treated by contracting

【现行译法】 consolidate what has come loose; Gathering the Dissipation; gathering the dispersed; treating dispersion with astringent

【推荐译法】 treat dissipation by astringing

【翻译说明】 "散"指耗散，译为 dissipation，而不是 dispersion（分散，

散开）或 loose（零散的；疏松的）。"收"指收涩，译为 astringe，而不是 gather（聚集）、contract（收缩）或 consolidate（使加强；合并）。为照顾术语的简洁性和类似术语结构的一致性，建议将"散者收之"译为 treat dissipation by astringing。

引例 Citations:

◎ 一曰酸收，泻下日久，则气散而不收，无能统摄，注泄何时而已？酸之一味，能助收肃之权，经云散者收之是也。（《冯氏锦囊秘录·杂症大小合参》卷五）

（一说酸味收敛，泄泻日久，使气散而不收敛，不能统摄，泄泻什么时候能好？酸味有助于收敛功能，这就是《黄帝内经》说的气血耗散的就予以收敛。）

There is a saying that sour taste is astringent. Prolonged diarrhea makes qi dissipate, unable to play its astringing and commanding role. How can diarrhea be cured? Sour taste helps with astringing. This is what is stated in *Huangdi's Inner Canon of Medicine*: "Treat dissipation by astringing." (*Feng's Secret Records in Brocade Bag*)

◎ 高者抑之，散者收之，治心肾神志不收者，法必本乎此。（《静香楼医案》三十一条）

（病势上盛上逆的就予以降逆抑制，气血耗散的就予以收敛，治疗心肾神志不能收敛的，方法必根源于这里。）

Treat excess in the upper and the adverse up-flow of qi by restraining and directing the counterflow of qi downward. Treat dissipation by astringing. They are surely fundamental to treating the non-astringent conditions related to the heart, kidney, and mind. (*Case Records of Jingxiang Mansion*) jīngzhě píng zhī

# 惊者平之

Treat Fright by Calming; Treat Fright by Exposure

惊者平之，中医治法之一，是指针对惊悸不安的病证，运用镇静安神的方药治疗。金代张从正将"惊者平之"引申为一种行为疗法，即对因感触异常之声像而患惊恐一类情志病，用常闻常见之法，使之适应而趋平静。从操作程序和方法上来看，与西方行为主义心理学的冲击疗法基本相同。

The term refers to a treatment method in traditional Chinese medicine. It means treating palpitations and fidgetiness with sedatives and tranquilizers. Zhang Congzheng of the Jin Dynasty developed the method of "treating fright by calming" into a behavioral therapy. He tried to familiarize patients with the abnormal sound or image that caused their emotional disorders such as fright by making them accustomed to it and stay calm. In this sense, it is called "treating fright with exposure therapy," which is essentially the same as the impact therapy of Western behaviorist psychology in terms of operating procedures and methods.

【曾经译法】 persons frightened should be calmed; tranquilizing the unease; frightened person should be calmed; fright is treated by calming; calming therapy for frightened disease

【现行译法】 relieving palpitation or convulsion with sedatives; relief of fright by calming; calm the one who takes fright; Relieve fright by tranquilization; Tranquilizing Palpitation; treating fright by calming; Calm him down when one is in terror; calm one who takes fright

【推荐译法】 1) treat fright by calming; 2) treat fright by exposure

【翻译说明】 "惊"指惊怯一类的情志病，译为 fright 较妥。palpitation 常表示"心悸"；convulsion 常表示"抽搐；痉挛"；terror 常表示"恐怖；惊骇"。"平"的本意是"使之平静"，译为clam（使平静），比 tranquilize（使安定；使镇静）更符合原意。后世将"平"也解释为"平常，习以为常"，引申出一种行为疗法，可借用西医词汇 exposure。为照顾术语的简洁性和类似术语结构的一致性，根据语境，"惊者平之"可译为 treat fright by calming 或者 treat fright by exposure。

引例 Citations:

◎ 惊者平之，平者常也。平常见之必无惊。（《儒门事亲·内伤形》）

（病属惊怯的可使人对外来刺激习以为常，平者，平常之义。平常见到的事物，肯定不会引起惊怯。）

Treat fright by exposure. Exposure means making one accustomed to the cause of fright so that it will no longer cause sudden fright. (*Confucians' Duties to Their Parents*) yǐ dú gōng dú

# 以毒攻毒

Counteract Poison with Poison

以毒攻毒，中医治法之一，即以药物的偏性特别是药物的毒副作用治疗由毒邪所致的病证。一般认为像恶性肿瘤、顽固的痈疽疮疡等一类病证，多由秽恶毒邪积蓄体内日久不化而成，非毒药不能攻之。如用蟾蜍之毒汁治疗乳癌、皮肤病、肝癌等，可收到较明显的疗效。但是，毒药毕竟有较大的毒副作用，临床用法、用量均应谨慎，也可通过改变剂型、提取有效成分或炮制以降低其毒性，或配合益气养血之药、甘缓平和之品以制约其毒性，以达到攻毒而不伤正的目的。

The term refers to a treatment method in traditional Chinese medicine. It means treating diseases caused by toxic pathogens with drastic medicinal properties, especially the toxic property of medicines. Diseases such as malignant tumors, protracted carbuncles, and sores are generally believed to be caused by the accumulation of pernicious and pathogenic factors, which can only be effectively removed by toxic agents. For example, toad venom can be used to treat breast cancer, skin disease, liver cancer, etc., all with marked therapeutic effects. Nevertheless, toxic agents do have significant side effects. Caution should be taken for their usage and dosage. The toxicity can be reduced by changing the forms of preparations, extracting effective ingredients, or using proper processing methods. Besides, medicines that can tonify qi and nourish blood, or sweet and mild-property ones, could be added to antagonize the toxicity, thus attacking poison without harming healthy qi.

【曾经译法】 treating the toxifying disease with poisonous agents; combating poison with poison; attacking toxin with toxin; treating virulent pathogen with poisonous agents

【现行译法】 treating the toxifying disease with poisonous agents; combating poison with poison/attacking toxin with toxin/using poison as an antidote for poison; treating the poisonous disease with poisonous agents; treating poison with poison; use of poisons as antidotes; counteracting poison with poison; fight poison with poison

【推荐译法】 counteract poison with poison

【翻译说明】 英语中表示"毒"的词主要有 poison 和 toxin。Poison 是统称，指可能造成伤害甚至导致死亡的毒物，大多源自自然。Toxin 偏指化学毒素。此术语中，"毒"不偏指化学毒素，译为 poison 较妥。英语中有 one's meat is another man's poison 的习语，可被译作"甲之熊掌，乙之砒霜"。相比 treat（治疗）、combat（战斗；防止）和 fight（战斗；打架），"攻"译为 counteract 较妥，表示"抵制；抵消；抵抗"。


引例 Citations:


◎ 盖斑蝥毒之尤者，虽曰以毒攻毒，惟少用之。(《景岳全书·古方八阵》)
　　(斑蝥毒性尤甚，虽说以毒攻毒，只能少量使用。)

Banmao (*Mylabris*, cantharide) is extremely toxic. It can be used to counteract poison; however, small dosage for use is the key. (*Complete Works of Jingyue*)

◎ 露蜂房，阳明药也，外科、齿科及他病用之者，亦皆取其以毒攻毒，兼杀虫之功焉。(《本草纲目·虫部》)
　　(露蜂房为阳明经药物，外科、牙科及其他疾病使用它，也都取它以毒攻毒兼杀虫的功效。)

*Lufengfang* (*Nidus Vespae*, honeycomb of paper wasps) is a medicine for the *yangming* meridian. It can be used for external, dental, and other diseases, all of which are based on its effects of counteracting poison with poison and killing worms. (*Compendium of Materia Medica*)

huǎnbǔ jígōng

# 缓补急攻

## Mild Tonification and Urgent Purgation

缓补急攻，中医治法之一，由于邪盛之实证——无论是外感或内生之邪，必然戕伐正气，且治疗时间越长，正气和脏腑功能受损越严重，甚或导致变证，故在使用攻法时，行动不能迟缓，应把握时机，迅速出击，及时截断扭转，杜绝病邪发展，彻底铲除病根，免生后患。而对于正虚的虚证，人体的正气恢复需要较长的时间，短时大补益并不能使气血的生成加快，况且患者脾胃虚弱，大宗进补还常有碍脾胃，阻滞运化，延缓气血的生成，非但无益，反而有害，所以补法不能贪求速效，只能缓图。

The term refers to a treatment method in traditional Chinese medicine. The excess patterns with exuberant pathogenic factors, whether being exogenous or endogenous, will result in the impairment of healthy qi. The longer the treatment duration is, the more damage it brings to healthy qi and *zang-fu* functions; or a deteriorated pattern may occur. Therefore, when purging method is to be used, timely action should be taken. Prompt treatment should be administered to reverse the development of disease in time, prevent it from progression, and eradicate its root cause without leaving any underlying risks. For deficiency patterns, it takes a relatively longer time for the body's healthy qi to recover. A short period of intense tonification cannot accelerate the supplementation of qi and blood. Moreover, patients with weak spleen and stomach cannot benefit directly from large tonifying formulas as tonics tend to bring burden to the spleen-stomach function, stagnate qi, and impede the production of qi and blood. Hence, tonification can only be planned for long-term outcomes, but not for immediate effects.

【曾经译法】无

【现行译法】无

【推荐译法】mild tonification and urgent purgation

【翻译说明】"补"指补益，可译为 tonification；"攻"指"攻下"，可译为 purgation。基于术语翻译的简洁性和类似术语结构的一致性，"缓补急攻"可译为 mild tonification and urgent purgation。

引例 Citations:

◎ 虚证如家贫室内空虚，铢铢累积，非旦夕间事，故无速法；实证如寇盗在家，开门急逐，贼去即安，故无缓法。(《医宗必读·辨治大法论》)

（虚证好像家里贫穷，屋内空虚，需要一点一滴地积累，不是短时间可以办到的事情，因此没有快速的办法；实证好像盗贼在家，开门赶快驱逐，盗贼离去就安宁，因此没有缓慢的办法。）

A deficiency pattern can be compared to an empty home due to poverty. It gradually develops and does not happen overnight, so urgent purgation is not recommended. An excess pattern is like a home occupied by an intruding burglar. The gate should be opened immediately to expel the housebreaker. Once the intruder is out, safety is restored, and so mild elimination is not recommended. (*Required Readings from the Medical Ancestors*)

◎ 病属于虚，宜治以缓……病属于实，宜治以急。(《神农本草经疏·治法提纲》)

（病属于虚证，治疗应缓慢……病属于实证，治疗应急速。）

If the disease is ascribed to a deficiency pattern, treatment should be mild. If the disease belongs to an excess pattern, urgent treatment is required. (*Commentary on "Shen Nong's Classic of Materia Medica"*) dàodì yàocái

# 道地药材

Geo-authentic Materia Medica

道地药材，又称地道药材，是优质纯正中药材的专用名词，指历史悠久、产地适宜、品种优良、产量宏丰、炮制考究、疗效突出、带有地域特点的中药材。天然药材的分布和生产离不开一定的自然条件。中国疆域辽阔，地貌复杂，涵盖北温带、寒温带、亚热带和热带，水土、日照、气候、生物分布等生态环境各地不尽相同，甚至南北差别很大，为各种药用动植物的生长和矿物的形成提供了有利的条件，同时也就使各种中药材的品种、产量和质量都有一定的地域性。古代医药学家经过长期使用、观察和比较发现，即便是分布较广的药材，也由于自然条件的不同，各地所产和质量优劣不一，逐渐形成了"道地药材"的概念。

The term refers to high-quality Chinese medicinal materials produced in a suitable area with a long cultivation history, excellent varieties, high yields, exquisite processing methods, marked therapeutic effects, and regional characteristics. The distribution and production of natural medicinal materials depend on certain natural factors. With a vast territory and complex geographical feature, China covers the north temperate zone, the cold temperate zone, the subtropical zone, and the tropical zone. Its ecological environment, such as water, soil, sunshine, climate, and biological distribution, tends to vary from place to place. Although the northern part of China is greatly different from its southern part, both provide favorable conditions for the formation of minerals and the growth of various medicinal animals and plants. They also bring them distinct regional characteristics, regardless of variety, yield, and quality. After a long period of use, observation, and comparison, ancient herbalists and healers had found that even the widely distributed medicinal materials were different in quality due to different natural conditions in different places; hence, the concept of "geo-authentic materia medica" gradually formed.

【曾经译法】 first-class drug; genuine regional drug

【现行译法】 genuine regional drug; genuine regional materia medica; authentic medicinal; authentic medicinal substances; geo-authentic materia medica

【推荐译法】 geo-authentic materia medica

【翻译说明】 前缀 geo- 表示"地球；土地；地理"等含义，"中药材"常译为 materia medica。"道地药材"是指在某一特定自然条件下和生态环境区域内产生的药材，建议译为 geo-authentic materia medica。以往译法中，genuine 侧重强调真假；authentic 与 genuine 是近义词，可以修饰形容食物，表示"地道的、正宗的"，例如 authentic Italian food（地道的意大利菜）。因此，采用 authentic 描述"道地药材"较妥。


引例 Citations:


◎ 选拣道地药材，务在精专，依方制度，心须殷勤。（《全幼心鉴》卷一）

（挑选道地药材，务必精专，按法炮制，用心必须周到。）


When preparing geo-authentic materia medica, whole-hearted attention should be paid to the technical details in selecting and processing. (*Mirror of Pediatric Treatment*)


◎ 如能照方预择道地药材，制好收贮，随时见症施治，利济无穷。（《古方汇精·凡例》）

（如果能够按照方剂事前选择道地药材，制好收藏，随时根据辨证施用，那么会获得无穷利益。）

If you choose geo-authentic materia medica according to the prescription, collect and prepare them in advance, and readily use them based on pattern differentiation, the benefits for patients will sustain. (*Essentials of Ancient Formulas*) páozhì

# 炮制

Processing of Medicines

炮制，古代又称"炮炙""修事""修治"等，是依据中医药理论，按照医疗、调配、制剂的不同要求以及药材自身性质，对中药所采取的加工处理技术。炮制是否得当对保证药效、用药安全、便于制剂和调剂都有十分重要的意义。由于中药材大都是生药，其中不少必须经过一定的炮制处理，才能符合临床用药的需要；有毒之品必须经过炮制后才能确保用药安全。按照不同的药性和治疗要求，中药有多种炮制方法，炮制的主要目的大致可以归纳为以下八个方面：①除去杂质，纯净药材；②切制饮片，便于调剂、制剂；③干燥药材，利于贮藏；④矫味、矫臭，便于服用；⑤降低毒副作用，保证安全用药；⑥增强药物功能，提高临床疗效；⑦改变药物性能，扩大应用范围；⑧引药入经，便于定向用药。

The term refers to processing Chinese medicinal materials according to the theories of traditional Chinese medicine, specifically according to different clinical, dispensing, and preparation needs as well as medicinal properties. Proper processing is of great significance to ensure efficacy, safety, convenience for preparation and dispensing. Because most Chinese medicinal materials are raw herbs, many of them must be processed to meet the needs of clinical use. Toxic agents must be processed for safety. Based on medicinal properties and treatment requirements, many processing methods are used, whose purposes can be roughly categorized into eight aspects: 1) removing unwanted matter to increase purity; 2) sizing medicinal materials to facilitate preparation; 3) drying medicinal materials to facilitate storage; 4) altering taste and smell to increase ease of ingestion; 5) reducing toxicity and side effects to ensure safety; 6) enhancing therapeutic function to achieve clinical efficacy; 7) changing medicinal properties to expand application, and 8) guiding the medicine to the target meridian.

【曾经译法】 process of preparing raw Chinese medicines (by roasting, baking, simmering, etc.); processing the drugs; preparation of crude medicines; processing drugs; herb processing; processing of medicinals; preparation (of medicinal herbs); drug processing; processing

【现行译法】 processing crude drugs; processing medicinal herbs; drug processing; Preparation of the herbs; Pao Zhi Preparation of Drugs; processing; preparing (herbal medicine); processing the drugs; processing of materia medica; preparation of crude drugs; herbal processing; processing (of materia medica); Processing

【推荐译法】 processing of medicines

【翻译说明】 Processing 本义为"加工（食品或原料）"。中药学中的"炮制"指的是通过一些加工方法用中草药原料制成药物的过程，即药物加工过程。2022 年发布的《世界卫生组织中医药术语国际标准》将之译为 processing of medicines。

引例 Citations:

◎ 京三棱……破积气，损真气，虚人勿用。火炮制使。（《本草发挥》卷二）

（京三棱……破积滞之气，损伤真气，体虚之人不要用。用火炮制使用。）

*Jingsanleng* (*Rhizoma Sparganii*, common burreed tuber) …, used to remove qi stagnation, will damage genuine qi, so patients with weak constitutions should avoid it. Fire processing before use is necessary. (*Elaboration on Materia Medica*)

◎ 虽曰据方炮制，对证投饵，其与实实虚虚、损不足补有余者何以异？
（《太平惠民和剂局方·叙意》）

　　（虽然说是根据处方要求炮制，对证用药，但与对实证用补法、
　　虚证用泻法者有什么差异？）

Although it is a rule that medicines should be processed according to prescription requirements and used based on pattern identification, what difference does it make when it comes to using tonifying method for excess patterns and using purgative method for deficiency patterns? (*Beneficial Formulas from the Taiping Imperial Pharmacy*) qīqíng héhé

# 七情和合

Seven Features of Compatibility

　　七情和合，是指药物配伍中的特殊关系，《神农本草经·序录》将各种药物的配伍关系概括为单行、相须、相使、相畏、相杀、相恶、相反等七个方面，统称为"七情和合"。凡不用其他药物辅助，单味药就可发挥作用者，称为"单行"。凡两种性能相宜的药物合用可以发生协同作用，称为"相须"。凡两种性能不同的药物合用，能互相促进，提高疗效，称为"相使"。凡两种药物合用，某一种药物能抑制另一种药物的烈性或毒性，称为"相畏"。凡一种药物能减轻或消除另一种药物的毒性或不良反应，称为"相杀"。凡两种药物合用，能相互牵制而使药效降低甚或消失，称为"相恶"。凡两种药物合用，可能发生不良反应或毒性作用，称为"相反"。相须、相使是中药配伍最常用的形式，相畏、相杀是不同程度的拮抗作用，相恶、相反属于配伍禁忌。

The term refers to the special patterns of combinations among Chinese medicines. A total of seven features were summarized in the Preface to *Shennong's Classic of Materia Medica* regarding the compatibility of various medicines, including the use of a single medicine, mutual reinforcement, mutual assistance, mutual restraint, mutual suppression, mutual aversion, and mutual opposition. When a medicine is used alone and there is no need to add another to assist it, it is called "single medicine." When two medicines of similar properties are used together, producing a synergistic effect, it is called "mutual reinforcement." When two medicines with different properties are used together to enhance each other's action and improve therapeutic effects, it is called "mutual assistance." When two medicines are used in combination and harsh effects or toxicity of one medicine can be restrained by the other, it is called "mutual restraint." When two medicines are used in combination and toxic or adverse effects of one medicine can be reduced or eliminated by the other, it is called "mutual suppression." When two medicines are used in combination and positive effects of one medicine can be counteracted and reduced or eliminated by the other, it is called "mutual aversion." When two medicines are used in combination and adverse reactions or toxicity may occur, it is called "mutual opposition." Mutual reinforcement and mutual assistance are the most commonly used forms of compatibility in traditional Chinese medicine. Mutual restraint and mutual suppression produce antagonistic effects of varying degrees. Mutual aversion and mutual opposition are contraindicated in terms of compatibility.

【曾经译法】 无

【现行译法】 无

【推荐译法】 seven features of compatibility

【翻译说明】 "七情和合" 是指将两味或两味以上的药配在一个方剂中。 "和合" 指药物配伍中的特殊关系, 有配伍、共存之意, 可译为 compatibility; "七情" 即有七种基本规律, 建议将 "七情和合" 译为 seven features of compatibility。


引例 Citation:


◎ 药有阴阳配合……有单行者, 有相须者, 有相使者, 有相畏者, 有相恶者, 有相反者, 有相杀者, 凡此七情, 合和视之。(《神农本草经·序例》)

(药性有阴阳配伍……有单行者, 有相须者, 有相使者, 有相畏者, 有相恶者, 有相反者, 有相杀者, 凡此七种情况, 应综合加以考察。)

There are yin and yang compatibilities of Chinese medicines... The seven features, i.e., single medicine, mutual reinforcement, mutual assistance, mutual restraint, mutual aversion, mutual opposition, and mutual suppression, should be comprehensively investigated. (*Shennong's Classic of Materia Medica*) guījīng

# 归经

## Meridian Tropism

归经是指药物对机体某部分的选择性作用，即某药对某些脏腑经络有特殊的亲和作用，因而对这些部位的病变起着主要或特殊的治疗作用。归经指明了药物治病的适用范围，是药物作用的定位概念。中药归经理论的形成是在中医基本理论指导下，以脏腑经络学说为基础、以药物所治疗的具体病证为依据，经过长期临床实践总结出来的用药理论。由于病变脏腑功能及经络循行部位不同，临床上所表现的症状各不相同。药物对相应的脏腑或者经络病变有治疗作用，就将这些脏腑或经络跟这些药物联系在一起。

The term refers to the selective effects of medicines on certain parts of the human body. Chinese medicines tend to have special affinities to some *zang-fu* organs and meridians, thus playing a major or special therapeutic role in treating these specific diseased areas. Meridian tropism theory pinpoints the indicated area of these medicines and their direction of actions. The theory has been developed through long-term clinical practice under the guidance of basic theories of traditional Chinese medicine, especially the *zang-fu* meridian theory. It is based on specific diseases and patterns treated by medicines. Due to different functions and locations of *zang-fu* organs and meridians, clinical manifestations are different. Medicines that go to specific *zang-fu* organs and meridians show targeted therapeutic effects, and they are thus associated with these *zang-fu* organs and meridians.

【曾经译法】 attributive channel (indicating a relationship between medicine and channel); channel-tropism; channel distribution (of medicines); channel tropism; meridian tropism; channel entry; meridian distribution (of drugs)

【现行译法】 meridian tropism; meridian distribution of drugs/channel distribution of medicines; channel entry; channel tropism; channel distribution; meridian distribution

【推荐译法】 meridian tropism

【翻译说明】 "归"，即"归属"，指药物作用的归属，说明药物作用对机体某部分的选择性。Tropism 意思是"向"，表示趋向性。"经"即人体的脏腑经络，可译为 meridian。建议将"归经"译为 meridian tropism。


引例 Citations:


◎ 桔梗……归经：入肺、心二经，兼入胃经，为开发和解之品。（《要药分剂》卷一）

> （桔梗……作用的脏腑经络部位：入肺、心二经，兼入胃经，是开发和解的药物。）

*Jiegeng* (*Radix Platycodonis*, platycodonroot)… enters the lung and the heart meridians, and also enters the stomach meridian. It is a dispersing and harmonizing agent. (*Classified Essential Materia Medica in Prescriptions*)

◎ 海藏则分肉桂、桂心、桂枝为三项，明其各有归经。（《要药分剂补正》卷十）

> （王海藏则分别肉桂、桂心、桂枝为三种，以明确三种药物各有不同的作用部位。）

Wang Haizang distinguished between three parts of cinnamon, i.e., *rougui* (*Cortex Cinnamomi*, cinnamon bark), *guixin* (*Cortex Cinnamomi*, inner bark of cinnamon), and *guizhi* (*Ramulus Cinnamomi*, cinnamon twig), to specify their different meridian tropism. (*Supplement to and Corrections on Classified Essential Materia Medica in Prescriptions*) yǐnjīngbàoshǐ

# 引经报使

Meridian-guiding Property

引经报使，又称引经，是中药的性能之一，指某些药物对某一脏腑经络有特殊作用，其选择性较强，并能引导其他药物的药力到达病变部位，从而提高临床疗效。从治疗意义上来说，主要是作为各经用药的向导，这类药物称为引经药。对引经报使和引经药的认识，是建立在归经理论基础之上的，是归经理论的重要组成部分。但归经只是针对某药本身而言，而引经报使则是归经与配伍的结合，引导相配伍的药物到达本经。引经药大体可分为十二经引经药、病证引经药以及局部穴位引经药三类。

The term refers to one of the properties of Chinese medicines. Some medicines have special effects on certain *zang-fu* organs and meridians and can guide other medicines to reach the affected meridians and body parts to improve therapeutic effects. They are thus called meridian-guiding medicines. The understanding of meridian-guiding property and meridian-guiding medicines is based on meridian tropism theory and is thus an important part of the latter. However, meridian tropism refers only to the direction of actions of a certain medicine, while meridian-guiding property is an integration of meridian tropism and medicine combinations to guide other ingredients of a formula to reach the target meridian. Meridian-guiding medicines are divided into three types: meridian-guiding medicines for the twelve meridians, meridian-guiding medicines for disease patterns, and meridian-guiding medicines for local acupoints.

【曾经译法】 medicinal guide; guiding drugs; guiding action; meridian guiding action; channel conduction; guiding medicinal herb

【现行译法】 meridian-guiding herb; directing to the affected meridian or site; Guiding action; guiding drugs; guiding action; medicinal guide; directing herbal actions to the diseased meridian or site; directing to the affected meridian/channel or site

【推荐译法】 meridian-guiding property

【翻译说明】 "引经报使"也称"引经"，是中药的一种性能，"引"即"引导"，选用 guide 较妥；"经"即人体的脏腑经络。"引经报使"可译为 meridian-guiding property。

引例 Citations:

◎ 引经报使……此皆引经之药，剂中用为向导，则能接引众药，直入本经，用力寡而获效捷也。(《本草洞诠》卷二十)

（引经报使……这些都是引经的药物，在方剂中作为向导，能引导众药，直接到达本经，用力少而获效快。）

Meridian-guiding property... These are meridian-guiding medicines. As the guides in a formula, they can guide other medicines directly to the target meridian in small doses, yet with a quick effect. (*Annotations on Materia Medica*)

◎ 头痛须用川芎，如不愈，各加引经药，太阳蔓荆，阳明白芷，少阳柴胡，太阴苍术，少阴细辛，厥阴吴茱萸。(《医学启源》卷上)

（头痛必须用川芎，如果不愈，应加用引经的药物，太阳经用蔓荆子，阳明经用白芷，少阳经用柴胡，太阴经用苍术，少阴经用细辛，厥阴经用吴茱萸。）

To treat headache, *chuanxiong* (*Rhizoma Chuanxiong*, Sichuan lovage rhizome) must be prescribed. If it is not cured, other meridian-guiding medicines should be added, such as *manjingzi* (*Fructus Viticis*, shrub chastetree fruit) for the *taiyang* meridian, *baizhi* (*Radix Angelicae Dahuricae*, angelica root) for the *yangming* meridian, *chaihu* (*Radix Bupleuri*, Chinese thorowax root) for the *shaoyang* meridian, *cangzhu* (*Rhizoma Atractylodis*, atractylodes rhizome) for the *taiyin* meridian, *xixin* (*Radix et Rhizoma Asari*, Manchurian wild ginger) for the *shaoyin* meridian, and *wuzhuyu* (*Fructus Evodiae*, medicine evodia fruit) for the *jueyin* meridian. (*The Origin of Medicine*)

# 十八反

Eighteen Antagonisms

十八反，中药配伍禁忌内容之一。所谓配伍禁忌，就是指某些中药合用会产生或增强剧烈的毒副作用或降低、破坏药效，因而应该避免配合应用。"十八反歌诀"最早见于金代张子和著《儒门事亲》，具体内容指乌头（包括川乌、草乌、附子）反浙贝母、川贝母、平贝母、伊贝母、湖北贝母、瓜蒌、瓜蒌皮、瓜蒌子、天花粉、半夏、白及、白蔹，甘草反甘遂、京大戟、红大戟、海藻、芫花，藜芦反人参、西洋参、党参、丹参、玄参、南沙参、北沙参、苦参、细辛、白芍、赤芍。但这些结论还有待进一步研究。

The term refers to the contraindicated combinations of Chinese medicines. Contraindicated combination means that the combination of some medicines will produce or enhance severe toxic or side effects, or reduce or minimize efficacy, and should all be avoided. The "rhymed verse of eighteen antagonisms" was first documented in the *Confucians' Duties to Their Parents* written by Zhang Zihe of the Jin Dynasty. The antagonisms include: *wutou* (*Radix Aconiti*, aconite) [including *chuanwu* (*Radix Aconiti*, common monkshood mother root), *caowu* (*Radix Aconiti Kusnezoffii*, kusnezoff monkshood root), and *fuzi* (*Radix Aconiti Lateralis Praeparata*, common monkshood branched root)] is antagonistic to *zhebeimu* (*Bulbus Fritillariae Thunbergii*, thunberg fritillary bulb), *chuanbeimu* (*Bulbus Fritillariae Cirrhosae*, Sichuan fritillary bulb), *pingbeimu* (*Bulbus Fritillariae Ussuriensis*, ussuri fritillay bulb), *yibeimu* (*Bulbus Fritillariae Pallidiflorae*, sinkiang fritillary bulb), *hubeibeimu* (*Bulbus Fritillariae Hupehensis*, hupeh fritillary bulb), *gualou* (*Fructus Trichosanthis*, snakegourd fruit), *gualoupi* (*Pericarpium Trichosanthis*, snakegourd peel), *gualouzi* (*Semen Trichosanthis*, snakegourd seed), *tianhuafen* (*Radix Trichosanthis*, snakegourd root), *banxia* (*Rhizoma Pinelliae*, pinellia rhizome), *baiji* (*Rhizoma Bletillae*, bletilla rhizome), and *bailian* (*Radix Ampelopsis*, ampelopsis); *gancao* (*Radix et Rhizoma Glycyrrhizae*, licorice root) is antagonistic to *gansui* (*Radix Kansui*, gansui root), *jingdaji* (*Radix Euphorbiae Pekinensis*, Peking euphorbia root), *hongdaji* (*Radix Knoxiae*, knoxia root), *haizao* (*Sargassum*, seaweed), and *yuanhua* (*Flos Genkwa*, lilac daphne flower bud); *lilu* (*Radix et Rhizoma Veratri Nigri*, veratrum root and rhizome) is antagonistic to *renshen* (*Radix et Rhizoma Ginseng*, ginseng), *xiyangshen* (*Radix Panacis Quinquefolii*, American ginseng), *dangshen* (*Radix Codonopsis*, codonopsis root), *danshen* (*Radix et Rhizoma Salviae Miltiorrhizae*, danshen root), *xuanshen* (*Radix Scrophulariae*, figwort root), *nanshashen* (*Radix Adenophorae*, four leaf ladybell root), *beishashen* (*Radix Glehniae*, coastal glehnia root), *kushen* (*Radix Sophorae Flavescentis*, light yellow sophora root), *xixin* (*Radix et Rhizoma Asari*, Manchurian wild ginger), *baishao* (*Radix Paeoniae Alba*, white peony root), and *chishao* (*Radix Paeoniae Rubra*, red peony root). However, these claims still need further investigation.

【曾经译法】 antagonism in the eighteen medicinal herbs; eighteen incompatibilities; antagonism among the eighteen medicinal herbs; eighteen incompatible medicaments; eighteen incompatible herbs; eighteen clashes; eighteen antagonisms

【现行译法】 eighteen incompatible medicaments; eighteen incompatible herbs/eighteen antagonisms; Eighteen incompatible medication; eighteen clashes; eighteen incompatibilities

【推荐译法】 eighteen antagonisms

【翻译说明】 "反"即不相容，是中药中的配伍禁忌，会产生严重副作用，antagonism 指"敌对"。建议将"十八反"译为 eighteen antagonisms。


引例 Citations:


◎ 本草名言十八反，半蒌贝蔹及攻乌，藻戟遂芫俱战草，诸参辛芍叛藜芦。（《儒门事亲》卷十四）

（中药学中著名的"十八反"，就是指半夏、瓜蒌、贝母、白蔹、白及与乌头相反，海藻、大戟、甘遂、芫花与甘草相反，人参、沙参、丹参、苦参、玄参、细辛、芍药与藜芦相反。）

The well-known eighteen antagonisms in Chinese medicines are as follows: *wutou* (*Radix Aconiti*, aconite) is antagonistic to *banxia* (*Rhizoma Pinelliae*, pinellia rhizome), *gualou* (*Fructus Trichosanthis*, snakegourd fruit), *beimu* (*Bulbus Fritillariae*, fritillary bulb), *bailian* (*Radix Ampelopsis*, ampelopsis), and *baiji* (*Rhizoma Bletillae*, bletilla rhizome); *gancao* (*Radix et Rhizoma Glycyrrhizae*, licorice root) is antagonistic to *haizao* (*Sargassum*, seaweed), *daji* (*Radix Euphorbiae Pekinensis seu Knoxiae*, Peking euphorbia root or knoxia root), *gansui* (*Radix Kansui*, gansui root), and *yuanhua* (*Flos Genkwa*, lilac daphne flower bud); *lilu* (*Radix et Rhizoma Veratri Nigri*, veratrum root and rhizome) is antagonistic to *renshen* (*Radix et Rhizoma Ginseng*, ginseng), *shashen* (Radix Adenophorae seu Glehniae, four leaf ladybell root or coastal glehnia root), *danshen* (*Radix et Rhizoma Salviae Miltiorrhizae*, danshen root), *kushen* (*Radix Sophorae Flavescentis*, light yellow sophora root), *xuanshen* (*Radix Scrophulariae*, figwort root), *xixin* (*Radix et Rhizoma Asari*, Manchurian wild ginger), and *shaoyao* (*Radix Paeoniae Alba seu Rubra*, white or red peony root). (*Confucians' Duties to Their Parents*)

◎ 十八反药性：人参芍药与沙参，细辛玄参及紫参，苦参丹参并前药，一见藜芦便杀人。白及白蔹并半夏，瓜蒌贝母五般真，莫见乌头与乌喙，逢之一反疾如神。大戟芫花并海藻，甘遂以上反甘草。（《药鉴》卷一）

> （十八反的药性：人参、芍药、沙参、细辛、玄参、紫参、苦参、丹参，以上药物与藜芦配伍就会杀人。白及、白蔹、半夏、瓜蒌、贝母五种药物，不能与乌头、乌喙合用，否则很快就会呈现毒副作用。大戟、芫花、海藻、甘遂，以上药物反甘草。）

The properties of medicines in the eighteen antagonisms are as follows: *Renshen* (*Radix et Rhizoma Ginseng*, ginseng), *shaoyao* (*Radix Paeoniae Alba seu Rubra*, white or red peony root), *shashen* (*Radix Adenophorae seu Glehniae*, four leaf ladybell root or coastal glehnia root), *xixin* (*Radix et Rhizoma Asari*, Manchurian wild ginger), *xuanshen* (*Radix Scrophulariae*, figwort root), *zishen* (*Herba Salviae Chinensis*, Chinese sage), *kushen* (*Radix Sophorae Flavescentis*, light yellow sophora root), and *danshen* (*Radix et Rhizoma Salviae Miltiorrhizae*, danshen root) are lethal when used together with *lilu* (*Radix et Rhizoma Veratri Nigri*, veratrum root and rhizome). *Wutou* (*Radix Aconiti*, aconite) and *wuhui* (*Radix Aconiti*, common monkshood root) are antagonistic to *baiji* (*Rhizoma Bletillae*, bletilla rhizome), *bailian* (*Radix Ampelopsis*, ampelopsis), *banxia* (*Rhizoma Pinelliae*, pinellia rhizome), *gualou* (*Fructus Trichosanthis*, snakegourd fruit), and *beimu* (*Bulbus Fritillariae*, fritillary bulb). When these combinations are used, toxic or side-effects will soon occur. *Gancao* (*Radix et Rhizoma Glycyrrhizae*, licorice root) is antagonistic to *daji* (*Radix Euphorbiae Pekinensis seu Knoxiae*, Peking euphorbia root or knoxia root), *yuanhua* (*Flos Genkwa*, lilac daphne flower bud), *haizao* (*Sargassum*, seaweed), and *gansui* (*Radix Kansui*, gansui root). (*Mirror of Medicinals*) shíjiǔwèi

# 十九畏

Nineteen Incompatibilities

十九畏，中药配伍禁忌内容之一。"十九畏歌诀"首见于明朝刘纯《医经小学》，十九畏的具体内容是指硫黄畏朴硝（芒硝），水银畏砒霜，狼毒畏密陀僧，巴豆畏牵牛，丁香畏郁金，川乌、草乌畏犀角，牙硝（芒硝）畏三棱，官桂（肉桂）畏赤石脂，人参畏五灵脂。这些结论还有待进一步研究。

The term refers to the contraindicated combinations of Chinese medicines. The "rhymed verse of nineteen incompatibilities" was first documented in *General Study on Medical Classics* written by Liu Chun of the Ming Dynasty. The nineteen incompatibilities are as follows: *liuhuang* (*Sulfur*, sulfur) is incompatible with *poxiao* or *mangxiao* (*Mirabilitum seu Natrii Sulfas*, mirabilite or sodium sulphate); *shuiyin* (*Hydrargyrum*, mercury) is incompatible with *pishuang* (*Arsenicum Sablimatum*, Arsenic); *langdu* (*Radix Euphorbiae Fischerianae*, wolf's bane) is incompatible with *mituoseng* (*Lithargyrum*, litharge); *badou* (*Semen Crotonis*, croton seed) is incompatible with *qianniu* (*Semen Pharbitidis*, pharbitidis seed); *dingxiang* (*Flos Caryophylli*, clove flower) is incompatible with *yujin* (*Radix Curcumae*, turmeric root tuber); *chuanwu* (*Radix Aconiti*, common monkshood mother root) and *caowu* (*Radix Aconiti Kusnezoffii*, kusnezoff monkshood root) are incompatible with *xijiao* (*Cornu Rhinocerotis*, rhinoceros horn); *yaxiao* or *mangxiao* (*Natrii Sulfas*, sodium sulphate) is incompatible with *sanleng* (*Rhizoma Sparganii*, common burreed tuber); *guangui* or *rougui* (*Cortex Cinnamomi*, cinnamon bark) is incompatible with *chishizhi* (*Halloysitum Rubrum*, halloysite); and *renshen* (*Radix et Rhizoma Ginseng*, ginseng) is incompatible with *wulingzhi* (*Faeces Trogopterori*, flying squirrel faeces). However, these claims still need further investigation.

【曾经译法】incompatibility in the nineteen medicinal herbs; nineteen antagonisms; mutual inhibition among the nineteen medicinal herbs; nineteen medicaments of mutual antagonism; nineteen herbs of mutual antagonism; nineteen fears; nineteen mutual inhibitions; nineteen medicaments of mutual antagonism; nineteen incompatibilities

【现行译法】 nineteen medicaments of mutual antagonism; nineteen inhibition/nineteen mutual antagonisms of herbs; nineteen incompatibilities; Nineteen medicaments of mutual restraint; nineteen antagonisms; nineteen mutual inhibitions

【推荐译法】 nineteen incompatibilities

【翻译说明】 "畏"指中药配伍禁忌，会减弱药效或者中和药效，相比"十八反"程度较轻。2022 年发布的《世界卫生组织中医药术语国际标准》将"十九畏"译为 nineteen incompatibilities。


引例 Citation:


◎ 又有十八反十九畏……所以畏者，硫黄与朴硝相畏。(《杏苑生春》卷一)

（另有用药禁忌的十八反与十九畏……所谓畏者，如硫黄与朴硝不宜合用。）

There are eighteen antagonisms and nineteen incompatibilities… Incompatibilities can be exemplified by the inappropriate combination of *liuhuang* (*Sulfur*, sulfur) and *poxiao* (*Mirabilitum seu Natrii Sulfas*, mirabilite). (*Spring in Apricot Woods*)

gāofāng

# 膏方

Medicated Paste

膏方，亦称膏剂，本指将药物用水或植物油煎熬浓缩而成的膏状剂型，有内服和外用两种。先秦至今，膏方大致经历了外用膏方、内服膏方、治疗范围扩大、着重于养生保健等多个阶段。现代所言膏方，多指内服用的煎膏，又称膏滋，是将具有调补阴阳、滋养润泽、强体补虚等综合作用的中药加水反复煎煮，去渣浓缩后，加炼蜜或炼糖制成的半液体剂型。其特点是药物浓度高、体积小、药效稳定、服用方便、口感好、便于携带等，一般用于慢性病虚弱的患者。如鹿胎膏、八珍益母膏等。

The term refers to a preparation form made from decocted medicines with water or vegetable oil, which can be taken orally or applied externally. Since the pre-Qin period, the development of medicated paste has roughly undergone several stages, from external use, oral use, extension of indications, to emphasis on health cultivation and disease prevention. In modern times, medicated paste mainly refers to the paste for oral administration. It is a semi-liquid form made from Chinese medicines with effects of tonifying yin and yang, nourishing and moistening, strengthening the body, and tonifying the deficiency. The medicines are repeatedly boiled in water until the decoction is condensed, and then dregs are removed and honey or sugar is added for processing. It is characterized by high concentration, small volume, stable efficacy, ease of ingestion, good taste, and convenience for one to carry. The paste is usually prescribed for patients with chronic disease and weakness, for example, *Lutai* Paste (Deer Placenta Paste) and *Bazhen Yimu* Paste (Eight-gem Motherwort Paste).

【曾经译法】无

【现行译法】paste; syrup; plaster

【推荐译法】medicated paste

【翻译说明】"膏方"指稠厚状半流质或冻状剂型的成药，可译为 medicated paste。

引例 Citations:

◎ 治虚冷枯瘦，身无精光，虚损诸不足，陆抗膏方：牛髓、羊脂各二升，白蜜、生姜汁、酥各三升。(《备急千金要方》卷十二)

    (治疗体虚怕冷，干枯消瘦，身体没有光彩，虚损各种不足，陆抗膏方：牛髓、羊脂各二升，白蜜、生姜汁、酥各三升。)

To treat constitutional weakness, fear of cold, emaciation, lack of luster, and other insufficiencies, use *Lu Kang* Paste. Its ingredients include beef bone marrow (two *sheng* or 400 ml), mutton fat (two *sheng* or 400 ml), white honey (three *sheng* or 600 ml), ginger juice (three *sheng* or 600 ml), and lard (three *sheng* or 600 ml). (*Important Formulas Worth a Thousand Gold Pieces for Emergency*)

◎ 凡属丸剂膏方，俗每以补益上品汇集成方。(《张聿青医案》卷二十)

    (凡是属于丸剂、膏方，习俗常用补益药物的上等药材汇集成方子。)

Formulas of pills or pastes usually consist of top-grade tonic medicines. (*Zhang Yuqing's Case Records*) língdān-miàoyào

# 灵丹妙药

Panacea; Magic Pill

灵丹妙药，原指有灵验效果的仙丹、能治百病的奇药，后用以比喻能够解决一切问题的办法。在中医学中，灵丹妙药更体现在对药物的经验总结和应用上。中医学有神农尝百草的传说，说明中医学所讲的"灵丹"，都是长期经验总结的结果，是临床疗效确切、作用机制明确的药物，如目前大家熟知的麝香保心丸、苏合香丸、安宫牛黄丸等。所谓"妙药"，除了药物本身的疗效外，其作用的发挥，还在于医生的使用方法、时机等。可能只是普通的一味中药，但如果辨证准确、配伍合理，就能够达到意想不到的效果，从而成为"妙药"。

The term refers to a pill with a miraculous effect that can cure various diseases. Nowadays, it is used as a metaphor for solutions to all problems. The term contains two parts of meaning as far as traditional Chinese medicine (TCM) is concerned. The first part "*lingdan* (灵丹, elixir)" describes the past drug-use experience. In TCM, there is a legend of Shennong tasting all kinds of herbs, which indicates that any panacea is the result of long-term experience based on definite clinical efficacy and the exact mechanism of action, such as the well-known *Shexiang Baoxin* Pill (Heart-protecting Musk Pill), *Suhexiang* Pill (Storax Pill), and *Angong Niuhuang* Pill (Peaceful Palace Bovine Bezoar Pill). The second part "*miaoyao* (妙药, wonder drug)" not only describes the efficacy of the medicine itself, but emphasizes the application, that is, how and when the doctor uses it. A medicine can be common; however, unexpectedly good outcomes may occur as a result of accurate pattern differentiation and rational combination with other medicines; then, it can be a "wonder drug."

【曾经译法】无

【现行译法】无

【推荐译法】panacea; magic pill

【翻译说明】采用归化策略，把"灵丹妙药"译为 panacea，便于西方读者理解。希腊神话中，帕那刻亚（Panakeia）是医药神阿斯库雷皮亚（Asclepius）的女儿，光明神阿波罗的孙女。帕那刻亚的名字在希腊语中是"治疗一切"的意思，由 pan + akeia 构成，相当于英语中的 all + cure。从她的名字衍生出英语单词 panacea，意思是"包治百病的灵丹妙药"。在口语等交际场景中，也可根据具体情况选择普通用语 magic pill。

引例 Citations:

◎ 今人不知其故，惊生地止血之神，视为灵丹妙药，日日煎服，久则脾胃太凉，必至泄泻。（《本草新编》卷一）

　　（现在的人不知道它的缘故，惊叹生地神奇的止血功效，将它视作灵丹妙药，每天煎服，日久会使脾胃过于寒凉，必然导致泄泻。）

People don't know why, but are amazed at the wonderful hemostatic effect of *shengdi* (*Radix Rehmanniae*, rehmannia root). They regard it as a panacea. But if it is taken every day, too much coldness will occur in the spleen and stomach and, as a result, will cause diarrhea. (*New Compilation of Materia Medica*)

◎ 我是天台一先生，逍遥散澹在心中。灵丹妙药都不用，吃的是生姜辣蒜大憨葱。（《瘸李岳诗酒玩江亭》第二折）

　　（我是天台山的一位先生，逍遥散淡在我心中。灵丹妙药都不用，吃的是生姜、大蒜与大葱。）

I am a gentleman living at ease and peace in Tiantanshan (a place in the present Zhejiang Province). No need of magic pills for me, but ginger, garlic, and green onions. (*Li Tieguai in the Pavilion by the River*)

# 对症下药

Suit the Remedy to the Case

对症下药，也称对证下药，是指医生针对病证开方用药。比喻针对具体情况、问题，提出具体的解决办法。典故出自《三国志·魏志·华佗传》：府吏倪寻和李延两人都患头痛发热，一同去请华佗诊治。华佗经过仔细望色、诊脉，开出两个不同的处方，交给患者取药回家煎服。两位患者一看处方，给倪寻开的是泻下药，而给李延开的是解表药。他们想：我俩症状相同，为什么开的药方却不同呢，是不是华佗弄错了？于是，他们向华佗请教。华佗解释道：倪寻的病是由于饮食过多引起的，病在内部，应当服泻下药，将积滞泻去．病就会好；李延的病是受凉感冒引起的，病在外部，应当吃解表药，风寒之邪随汗而去，头痛也就好了。两人听了，十分信服，便回家将药熬好服下，果然很快都痊愈了。中医强调辨证论治，虽然所患疾病相同，但所表现的证不同，则用不同的方药治疗。

The term, also known as prescribing specific medicines for a pattern or syndrome, refers to a doctor prescribing medicines based on pattern diagnosis. Figuratively, it means that specific proper measures should be taken to solve specific problems. This phrase comes from the "Biography of Hua Tuo" in *Records of the Three Kingdoms*. The government officials Ni Xun and Li Yan both suffered from headaches and fever and went to see Hua Tuo for treatment. After carefully examining the complexion and feeling the pulse, Hua Tuo wrote two different prescriptions and asked them to take the medicines home for decoction. When they looked at the prescriptions, they found that Ni Xun received a purgative formula, while Li Yan was given an exterior-releasing one. "We both have the same symptoms. Why are the prescriptions different? Was Hua Tuo wrong?" So they asked Hua Tuo about this. Hua Tuo explained that Ni Xun's disease was caused by excessive food accumulation, which was endogenous, so he should take purgative medicines to eliminate food stagnation, and the disease would be cured. Li Yan was diagnosed with a cold. The disease was exogenous, so he should take exterior-releasing medicines. The wind and cold pathogens would go away with sweating, and the headache would be cured. They were convinced. Then they went back home and took the decoction of medicines. Soon enough, both of them regained health. Traditional Chinese medicine emphasizes treatment based on pattern differentiation. Although the manifestations are the same, the patterns are different, and different prescriptions should be used for treatment to suit the remedy to the case.

【曾经译法】 suit the medicine to the illness; suit the remedy to the case; prescribe specific medicine for illness; prescribing specific medicine for an illness; prescribing specific medicine based on concrete condition

【现行译法】 symptomatic treatment/expectant treatment; administering specific medications for an illness; suit the remedy to the case

【推荐译法】 suit the remedy to the case

【翻译说明】 "症"指"症状","证"即医生诊断出来的病证。"对症下药"指医生根据患者症状表现进行具体诊断后开方给药。目前此术语内涵已经扩大，常指根据具体情况，采取具体的解决问题的方法。因此，建议译为习语 suit the remedy to the case，便于理解。


引例 Citations:


◎ 克己复礼，便是捉得病根，对症下药。(《朱子语类》卷四十一)
　　(约束自我，使言行合乎先王之礼，就是抓住了病根，针对具体病证开方用药。)


Restraining yourself and making your words and deeds conform to the prescribed etiquette are just like seizing the root cause of the disease and suiting the remedy to the case. (*Thematic Discourses of Master Zhu*)

◎ 汗不出而烦躁，宜大青龙以发汗，对证下药，尤为的确。（《伤寒论集注》卷一）

（没有汗出而烦躁，应该用大青龙汤发汗，针对具体病证开方用药，尤为完全正确。）

For vexation with no sweating, *Da Qinglong* Decoction (Major Bluegreen Dragon Decoction) should be used to induce sweating. This is suiting the remedy to the case, and is absolutely correct. (*Collected Commentaries on "Treatise on Cold Damage"*) shí'èr jīngmài

# 十二经脉

Twelve Meridians

十二经脉，指十二脏腑所属的经脉，是经络系统的主体，也称为十二脉、十二经、十二正经等。十二经脉的名称由手足、阴阳、脏腑三部分组成。用手、足将十二经脉分成手六经和足六经，属六脏循于肢体内侧的经脉为阴经，属六腑循于肢体外侧、后面的经脉为阳经。阴阳又划分为三阴三阳，三阴为太阴、少阴、厥阴，三阳为阳明、太阳、少阳。基于上述命名原则，十二经脉的名称分别为手太阴肺经、手阳明大肠经、足阳明胃经、足太阴脾经、手少阴心经、手太阳小肠经、足太阳膀胱经、足少阴肾经、手厥阴心包经、手少阳三焦经、足少阳胆经、足厥阴肝经。

The term refers to the meridians of the twelve *zang-fu* organs, which is the principal part of the meridian system. The naming of the twelve meridians consists of hand-foot, yin-yang, and *zang-fu* organs. The twelve meridians are divided into the six meridians of the hand and the six meridians of the foot. The meridians that belong to the six *zang*-organs and flow along the medial side of the limbs are yin meridians; the meridians that belong to the six *fu*-organs and distribute along the lateral and posterior sides of the limbs are yang meridians. Yin and yang meridians are further divided into three yin and three yang meridians. The three yin are *taiyin*, *shaoyin* and *jueyin;* the three yang are *yangming*, *taiyang* and *shaoyang*. Based on the above principles, the names of the twelve meridians are as follows: the Lung Meridian of Hand-*taiyin*, the Large Intestine Meridian of Hand-*yangming*, the Stomach Meridian of Foot-*yangming*, the Spleen Meridian of Foot-*taiyin*, the Heart Meridian of Hand-*shaoyin*, the Small Intestine Meridian of Hand-*taiyang*, the Bladder Meridian of Foot-*taiyang*, the Kidney Meridian of Foot-*shaoyin*, the Pericardium Meridian of Hand-*jueyin*, the *Sanjiao* (Triple Energizer) Meridian of Hand-*shaoyang*, the Gallbladder Meridian of Foot-*shaoyang*, and the Liver Meridian of Foot-*jueyin*.

【曾经译法】 twelve channels; twelve regular channels; twelve regular meridians; twelve meridians

【现行译法】 twelve regular meridians; twelve meridians/twelve channels; Twelve Meridians; twelve main meridians; twelve regular channels

【推荐译法】 twelve meridians

【翻译说明】 "十二经脉"也称为"正经",译为 twelve meridians。此术语的翻译目前已经较为规范。


引例 Citations:


◎ 夫十二经脉者,内属于腑脏,外络于肢节。(《灵枢·海论》)

（十二经脉,在内连于五脏六腑,在外连于四肢关节。）

The twelve meridians are connected to the *zang-fu* organs internally and to the limbs and joints externally. (*Miraculous Pivot*)


◎ 地有十二经水,人有十二经脉……此人与天地相应者也。(《灵枢·邪客》)

（地上有十二条大河流,人体有十二条经脉……这些就是人体与天地相应的具体情况。）

There are twelve great rivers on the earth and twelve meridians in the human body. ... These are the specific conditions of the human body corresponding to nature. (*Miraculous Pivot*)

qíjīng bāmài

# 奇经八脉

Eight Extra Meridians

奇经八脉，是督脉、任脉、冲脉、带脉、阴跷脉、阳跷脉、阴维脉、阳维脉的总称。由于其分布不如十二经脉那样有规律，与脏腑没有直接的相互络属关系，相互之间也没有表里关系，有异于十二正经，故曰"奇经"。因其数有八，故称为"奇经八脉"。奇经八脉纵横交叉于十二经脉之间，能加强十二经脉之间联系，调节十二经脉气血，与脑、髓、女子胞等奇恒之腑以及肝、肾等脏联系密切。

The term refers to the eight meridians including the governor vessel, conception vessel, thoroughfare vessel, belt vessel, *yinqiao* meridian, *yangqiao* meridian, *yinwei* meridian, and *yangwei* meridian. Because their distributions are not as regular as those of the twelve meridians and there is no direct connecting relationship with the *zang-fu* organs and no exterior-interior relationship between each other, they are different from the twelve regular meridians, hence the name "extra meridians." As there are eight of them, they are called "the eight extra meridians." The eight extra meridians connect the twelve meridians. They strengthen the connection of the twelve meridians, regulate their qi and blood, and are closely related to the brain, marrow, uterus, as well as the liver, kidney, and other organs.

【曾经译法】 eight extra-channels; eight extra channels; eight extra-meridians; eight extraordinary vessels; Eight Extra-channels; eight extraordinary channels/meridians

【现行译法】 eight extra-meridians/eight extraordinary meridians; eight extraordinary vessels/eight extra-meridians/eight extra-vessels; eight extra meridians; Eight extra channels; eight extraordinary channels; eight extra channels

【推荐译法】 eight extra meridians

【翻译说明】针灸经络和穴位术语的翻译目前已经非常规范，遵循世界卫生组织总部针灸穴名国际标准化科学组会议审定通过的《标准针灸穴名》，"奇经八脉"翻译为 eight extra meridians，而"奇恒之腑"翻译为 extraordinary organs，以示区别。

引例 Citations:

◎ 脉有奇经八脉者，不拘于十二经，何也？然：有阳维，有阴维，有阳跷，有阴跷，有冲，有督，有任，有带之脉。凡此八脉者，皆不拘于经，故曰奇经八脉也。(《难经·二十七难》)

（经脉有奇经八脉，不限于十二经脉，为什么？回答说：有阳维、阴维、阳跷、阴跷、冲脉、督脉、任脉、带脉，凡是这八脉，都不限于十二经脉，因此，称为"奇经八脉"。）

There are eight extra meridians that are not pertaining to the twelve meridians. What are they? They are the *yangwei* meridian, *yinwei* meridian, *yangqiao* meridian, *yinqiao* meridian, thoroughfare vessel, governor vessel, conception vessel, and belt vessel. These eight meridians are different from the twelve regular meridians. As a result, they are called "the eight extra meridians." (*Canon of Difficult Issues*)

◎ 十二经者，常脉也。奇经八脉，则不拘于常，故谓之奇经。(《圣济总录》卷一百九十二)

（十二经脉是恒常之脉，奇经八脉则不限于恒常的范围，因此称为"奇经"。）

The twelve meridians are regular meridians; the eight extra meridians are out of this range. Hence, they are called "the extra meridians." (*Comprehensive Records of Sacred Benevolence*) shíwǔ luò

# 十五络

## Fifteen Collaterals

十五络，又称为"十五别络"，是指十二经之络，任脉、督脉之络，以及脾之大络在内的十五条络脉。十五络是从经脉分出的支脉，大多分布于体表，对全身无数细小的络脉起着主导作用。从别络分出的细小络脉称为"孙络"，分布在皮肤表面的络脉称为"浮络"。十五络的作用主要是加强十二经脉表里两经在体表的联系，以及人体前、后、侧面的统一联系，以灌渗气血，濡养全身。

The term refers to the fifteen collaterals including the collaterals of the twelve meridians, the collaterals of the governor vessel and the conception vessel, as well as the major collateral of the spleen. The fifteen collaterals are the branches separated from the meridians, which are mostly distributed on the surface of the body and play a leading role in numerous minor collaterals throughout the body. The extremely small collaterals separated from the fifteen collaterals are called "minute collaterals," and the collaterals distributed on the surface of the skin are called "floating collaterals." The functions of the fifteen collaterals are mainly to strengthen the exterior-interior connection of the twelve meridians on the surface of the body and enhance the unity of the front, back, and sides of the human body to supply qi and blood and nourish the whole body.

【曾经译法】 fifteen luos; fifteen largest collaterals; fifteen collateral channels; fifteen main collaterals; fifteen collaterals; fifteen network vessels

【现行译法】 fifteen collaterals; fifteen main collaterals; Fifteen Connecting Collaterals; fifteen collateral channels; fifteen collateral vessels

【推荐译法】 fifteen collaterals

【翻译说明】 针灸经络和穴位术语的翻译目前已经非常规范，遵循世界卫生组织总部针灸穴名国际标准化科学组会议审定通过的《标准针灸穴名》，"络脉"一般翻译为 collaterals。

引例 Citations:

◎ 凡此十五络者，实则必见，虚则必下。视之不见，求之上下，人经不同，络脉异所别也。（《灵枢·经脉》）

　　（上述十五条络脉，邪气实则络脉充盈可以看见，正气虚则络脉陷下而不易看见。如果在外表看不见，可在络脉上下寻求。由于每个人的经脉不同，络脉也有差异。）

The fifteen collaterals mentioned above can be detected when there is excess. When healthy qi is deficient, the collaterals sink and are not easy to identify. If they cannot be detected from the outside, they can be searched from the upper or lower part of the route. Collaterals also vary from person to person because each person has different meridians. (*Miraculous Pivot*)

◎ 十二经共十二络，而外有任督之络，及脾之大络，是为十五络也。（《类经·经络类》）

　　（十二经脉共有十二条络脉，另外有任脉、督脉的络脉，以及脾的大络，这就是十五络脉。）

There are twelve collaterals pertaining to the twelve meridians. With the collaterals of the conception vessel and the governor vessel, as well as the major collateral of the spleen, there are a total of fifteen collaterals. (*Classified Classics*)

# 十二经别

Twelve Divergent Meridians

十二经别，是十二经脉的表里关系形式，即四肢内外两侧对应分布的阴阳经脉，在走向躯干的过程中相合而行，阳脉合于阴脉而内联脏腑，阴脉合于阳脉而上行头面颈项，构成六对表里关系，以表达表里经脉共有的头身作用规律。每一对相为表里的经别组成一"合"，十二经别手足三阴三阳共组成六对，又称为"六合"。由于十二经别可分布到十二正经所未到之处，不仅使十二经脉分布和联系的部位更加周密，而且也相应扩大了十二经脉穴位的主治范围。

The term refers to the branches of the twelve meridians forming exterior-interior relationships. Distributed on the medial and lateral sides of the limbs, yin and yang meridians run in opposite directions towards the center of the torso. Yang meridians connect yin meridians, and vice versa. Accordingly, yang meridians link with the internal organs and yin meridians ascend to the head, face, and neck. Six pairs of branches with exterior-interior relationships enable the meridians to act on the head and body. Each pair is called one "*he*" (合, combination). Six yin meridians and six yang meridians of the hand and the foot make a total of six pairs, called "six combinations." The twelve divergent meridians facilitate closer distribution and connection of the twelve meridians and expand the indications of the acupoints as they can be distributed further than the twelve meridians.

【曾经译法】 internal branches of twelve channels; the branches of the twelve channels; branches of the twelve regular channels; twelve divergent meridians; twelve channel divergences; branches of twelve meridians; branches of twelve regular channels; branches of the twelve meridians

【现行译法】 branches of the twelve regular meridians; branches of twelve meridians/divergences of twelve meridians; twelve divergent meridians; Twelve Branches; the branches of the twelve channels; twelve meridian/channel divergences; twelve meridian divergences; internal branches of twelve channels

【推荐译法】 twelve divergent meridians

【翻译说明】 针灸经络和穴位术语的翻译目前已经非常规范，遵循世界卫生组织总部针灸穴名国际标准化科学组会议审定通过的《标准针灸穴名》。"经别"即指十二经的别支，故采用 twelve divergent meridians，而不是 twelve meridian divergences。

引例 Citations:

◎ 十二大经，复有正别。正，谓六阳大经别行，还合腑经。别，谓六阴大经别行，合于腑经，不还本经，故名为别。(《太素》卷九)

（十二经脉，又有正与别。正，指六条阳经别行，复会合于六腑经脉。别，指六条阴经别行，会合于相表里的六腑经脉，不返回本条经脉，因此称为"别"。）

For twelve meridians, there are regular and divergent ones. "Regular" means that six yang meridians are divided into branches and then return to the six meridians of *fu*-organs. "Divergent" means that six yin meridians are divided into branches, connecting six meridians of *fu*-organs, and do not return. (*Grand Simplicity*)

◎ 十二经脉与经别多过于此，即不然，亦在其前后左右也。(《医灯续焰》卷七)

（十二经脉与十二经别，多经过喉咙这个地方，即使不经过，也在喉咙的前后左右。）

The twelve meridians and their divergent branches often pass through the throat. Even if they do not pass through it directly, they are around it. (*Reburning the Lamp of Medicine*)

shí'èr jīngjīn

# 十二经筋

## Twelve Meridian Sinews

十二经筋，是十二经脉连属于肢体外周的筋膜（肌腱、韧带）、肌肉体系。依据十二经脉的分布，全身筋肉体系分为十二个部分，称为"十二经筋"。经筋有起、结、聚、布等分布特点，其走行方向均起于四肢末端，终止于头面躯干，分布区域大致与同名经脉的体表线路相吻合。经筋的主要作用是约束骨骼，有利于关节的屈伸运动。

The term refers to the fasciae (tendons, ligaments) and muscles around the limbs that are connected with the twelve meridians. Based on the distribution of the twelve meridians, the fascia and muscle system of the whole body is divided into twelve parts, which are called the twelve meridian sinews. They have the distribution characteristics of starting, ending, gathering, and distributing. All of them start from the end of extremities and end in the head, face, or torso, with the distribution area that matches the surface route of the corresponding meridian. The twelve meridian sinews control bones, facilitating the flexion and extension of joints.

【曾经译法】 tendons of the twelve channels; musculature of the twelve channels; muscles along the twelve regular channels; twelve meridian tendons; twelve channel sinews; musculature of twelve meridians

【现行译法】 twelve muscle regions, muscle along the twelve regular meridians; tendons of twelve meridians/sinews of twelve meridians; muscles along the twelve meridians; Twelve Muscular Regions; muscles along twelve meridians; musculature of the twelve channels; tendons along twelve meridians; twelve meridian/channel sinews; twelve meridian regions

【推荐译法】 twelve meridian sinews

【翻译说明】针灸经络和穴位术语的翻译目前已经非常规范，遵循世界卫生组织总部针灸穴名国际标准化科学组会议审定通过的《标准针灸穴名》，"十二经筋"译为 twelve meridian sinews。

引例 Citations:

◎ 十二经筋皆起于手足指，循络于身也。（《诸病源候论》卷二十二）

（十二经筋都起始于手足指，循行络于身体。）

The twelve meridian sinews start from the fingers or toes and circulate throughout the body. (*Treatise on the Causes and Manifestations of Various Diseases*)

◎ 十二经筋与十二经脉俱禀三阴三阳，行于手足，故分为十二。（《太素》卷十三）

（十二经筋与十二经脉，都具有三阴三阳的属性，循行于手足，因此分为十二条。）

There are twelve meridian sinews and twelve meridians as they both have the attributes of three yin and three yang, running from the hands or feet. (*Grand Simplicity*) shí'èr píbù

# 十二皮部

## Twelve Cutaneous Regions

十二皮部是指体表的皮肤按经络的分布部位分区。十二经脉及其所属络脉，在体表有一定的分布范围，与之相应，全身的皮肤也就划分为十二个部分，称为"十二皮部。"《素问·皮部论》云："欲知皮部，以经脉为纪。"因此，皮部就是十二经脉及其所属络脉在体表的分区，也是十二经脉之气的散布所在。皮部作为十二经脉的体表分区，与经脉、络脉的不同之处在于：经脉呈线状分布，络脉呈网状分布，而皮部则侧重于"面"的划分，其分布范围大致上属于该经循行的部位，而且比经络更为广泛。

The term refers to different parts of the skin along the distribution of the meridians and collaterals. The twelve meridians and their subordinate collaterals have their corresponding distribution areas on the body surface. Accordingly, the skin is also divided into twelve parts, called the twelve cutaneous regions. It is written in "The Theory of Skin" of *Plain Conversation* that meridians should be used as the principle of division to know the division of the skin. Therefore, the cutaneous regions are the division of the twelve meridians and their subordinate collaterals on the body surface, and also the place where the qi of the twelve meridians is distributed. As the division of the twelve meridians on the body surface, the cutaneous regions are different from the meridians and collaterals in that the meridians are distributed in a linear way and the collaterals are distributed in a network way. By contrast, the cutaneous regions cover the area that belongs to the corresponding meridians and is wider than that of the meridians and collaterals.

【曾经译法】 skin areas of the twelve channels; twelve cutaneous regions; twelve skin areas; twelve skin regions; twelve skin divisions

【现行译法】 twelve skin areas; twelve skin divisions; twelve cutaneous regions; The twelve skin zones; twelve skin regions; twelve body surface areas

181

【推荐译法】twelve cutaneous regions

【翻译说明】针灸经络和穴位术语的翻译目前已经非常规范，遵循世界卫生组织总部针灸穴名国际标准化科学组会议审定通过的《标准针灸穴名》，"皮部"的译文使用 cutaneous 而不是 skin，凸显医学专业术语的特征。

引例 Citations:

◎ 因视其皮部有血络者，尽取之。（《素问·缪刺论》）

（要看其皮部是否有瘀血的络脉，若有应将瘀血全部刺出来。）

It is necessary to examine whether there are collaterals with blood stasis in the cutaneous region. If so, the blood stasis should all be removed with acupuncture therapy. (*Plain Conversation*)

◎ 皮之十二部，其生病皆何如？（《素问·皮部论》）

（十二皮部，它们发病的情况是怎样的？）

How do diseases develop in the twelve cutaneous regions? (*Plain Conversation*) shí'èr jīng zhī hǎi

# 十二经之海

Sea of the Twelve Meridians

　　十二经脉之海，比喻冲脉在经脉中血气最为充盛。冲脉是奇经八脉之一，与督、任二脉一同起于胞中，下出会阴，从气街部起与足少阴经相并，与督脉相通，同足阳明经交会，上行于头，下至于足，后行于背，前布于胸腹，贯穿全身，通受十二经之气血，是总领诸经气血之要冲，调节十二经之气血，故称为"十二经之海"。

The term refers to the thoroughfare vessel which, among the meridians, contains the most abundant blood and qi. The thoroughfare vessel is one of the eight extra meridians. It starts from the uterus together with the governor vessel and the conception vessel, and goes down to the perineum. It runs in parallel with the Kidney Meridian of Foot-*shaoyin* from the qi pathway, connects the governor vessel, and intersects with the Stomach Meridian of Foot-*yangming*. It goes up to the head, down to the feet, backward to the back, and forward to the chest and abdomen, and thus runs through the whole body. It receives the qi and blood of the twelve meridians and regulates them, and is the important hub of all meridians. Therefore, it is called "the sea of the twelve meridians."

【曾经译法】 sea of the twelve channels (chong channel); the sea of the twelve regular channels; sea of the twelve meridians; sea of the twelve channels [the penetrating vessel]; thoroughfare vessel (meridian), TV

【现行译法】 sea of the twelve meridians; sea of twelve meridians/thoroughfare vessel; the sea of the twelve regular channels; reservoir of twelve meridians; reservoir of the twelve meridians

【推荐译法】 sea of the twelve meridians

【翻译说明】 建议将"十二经之海"译为 sea of the twelve meridians，保留术语的含义和特色。

引例 Citations:

◎ 冲脉者，为十二经之海，其输上在于大杼，下出于巨虚之上下廉。（《灵枢·海论》）

（冲脉是十二经之海，它的输注要穴，上在大杼，下在上巨虚与下巨虚。）

The thoroughfare vessel is the sea of the twelve meridians. Its infusion points are located at *dazhu* (BL11), the upper *juxu* (ST37), and the lower *juxu* (ST39). (*Miraculous Pivot*)

◎ 冲脉起于会阴，夹脐而行，直冲于上，为诸脉之冲要，故曰十二经脉之海。（《频湖脉学》）

（冲脉起始于会阴部位，夹脐而一直上行至口唇，是各脉的冲要，因此称为"十二经脉之海"。）

The thoroughfare vessel starts from the perineum, passes through the navel, and continues up to the lips. It is strategically important for each meridian, hence the name "the sea of the twelve meridians." (*Binhu's Sphygmology*) yángmài zhī hǎi

# 阳脉之海

Sea of Yang Meridians

阳脉之海，比喻督脉总督一身的阳经，调节全身阳经气血的作用。督脉为奇经八脉之一，行于背部正中，多次与手、足三阳经及阳维脉交会，是阳脉之总纲，有统率阳经和调节一身阳气的作用，故称为"阳脉之海"。

The term refers to the governor vessel which regulates the qi and blood of yang meridians. The governor vessel is one of the eight extra meridians, which runs in the middle of the back and intersects with the three yang meridians of the hand and the foot and the *yangwei* meridian. It governs yang meridians and has the function of regulating the yang qi of the whole body, hence the name "the sea of yang meridians."

【曾经译法】 sea of yang channels (du channel); the sea of the yang channels; the sea of yang meridians; sea of the yang vessels [the governing vessel]; governing vessel (meridian), GV; sea of yang channel

【现行译法】 sea of the yang meridian; sea of yang meridians/governor vessel; sea of Yang Channels; the sea of the yang channels; reservoir of yang meridians; reservoir of the yang meridians

【推荐译法】 sea of yang meridians

【翻译说明】 建议将"阳脉之海"译为 sea of yang meridians，保留术语的含义和特色。

引例 Citations:

◎ 督脉起于会阴，循背而行于身之后，为阳脉之总督，故曰阳脉之海。

（《奇经八脉考·八脉》）

（督脉起始于会阴部位，循背部上行于身体后面，是阳脉的总督，
因此称为"阳脉之海"。）

The governor vessel starts from the perineum and goes up along the back.
It governs yang meridians, hence the name "the sea of yang meridians."
(*Consideration of the Eight Extra Meridians*)

◎ 以人之脉络，周流于诸阳之分，譬犹水也，而督脉则为之都纲，故曰
阳脉之海。（《医旨绪余》卷下）

（由于人的脉络气血，像水一样周流在各阳经部分，而督脉是阳
经的都纲，因此称为"阳脉之海"。）

Qi and blood of meridians and collaterals flow around yang meridians like
water. The governor vessel governs yang meridians, and is called "the sea of
yang meridians." (*Remnants of Medical Decree*)

yīnmài zhī hǎi

# 阴脉之海

Sea of Yin Meridians

  阴脉之海，比喻任脉总任一身的阴经，调节全身阴经气血的作用。任脉为奇经八脉之一，行于腹胸正中线，其脉多次与足三阴经及阴维脉交会，能加强阴经之间的相互联系，调节一身阴经的气血，故称为"阴脉之海"。

The term refers to the conception vessel which regulates the qi and blood of yin meridians. The conception vessel is one of the eight extra meridians, which runs in the midline of the abdomen and chest and intersects with three yin meridians of the foot and the *yinwei* meridian. It can strengthen the connection and regulate the qi and blood of yin meridians, hence the name "the sea of yin meridians."

【曾经译法】 sea of yin channels (ren channel); the sea of the yin channels; the sea of yin meridians; sea of the yin vessels [conception vessel]; conception vessel (meridian); sea of yin channel

【现行译法】 sea of the yin meridian; sea of yin meridians (conception vessel); sea of Yin Channels, sea of Yin Meridians; the sea of the yin channels; reservoir of yin meridians

【推荐译法】 sea of yin meridians

【翻译说明】 此术语为字面翻译，保留术语的含义和特色。

  引例 Citations:

◎ 任脉起于会阴，循腹而行于身之前，为阴脉之承任，故曰阴脉之海。（《奇经八脉考·八脉》）

（任脉起始于会阴部，循腹部前正中线上行，总揽人体属阴的经脉，因此称为"阴脉之海"。）

The conception vessel starts from the perineum and goes up along the central line in the front of the body. It governs yin meridians of the human body, hence the name "the sea of yin meridians." (*Textual Research on the Eight Extra Meridians*)

◎ 以人之脉络，周流于诸阴之分，譬犹水也，而任脉则为之总会焉，故曰阴脉之海。（《医旨绪余》卷下）

（由于人的脉络气血，像水一样周流在各阴经部分，而任脉是阴经的总会，因此称为"阴脉之海"。）

Qi and blood of meridians and collaterals flow around yin meridians like water. The conception vessel is the gathering point of yin meridians, and is called "the sea of yin meridians." (*Remnants of Medical Decree*)

# 经穴

Meridian Points; *Jing* (River) Points

经穴，指归属于十二经脉或十二经脉与督脉、任脉上的腧穴的总称。另外，也指十二经脉上井、荥、输、经、合五输穴中的经穴。

It is a collective term for the acupoints pertaining to the twelve meridians, or for the acupoints on the twelve meridians, the governor vessel, and the conception vessel. In addition, it is used to refer to one type of the five transport points, namely *jing* (well) points, *ying* (spring) points, *shu* (stream) points, *jing* (river) points, and *he* (sea) points.

【曾经译法】 jing point; the jing (river) points; Jing points, the River points; 1) meridian points, 2) Jing-River points; river point [one of the five transport points]; channel point; acupoint; 1) points, 2) the Jing or River points; jing-river point; meridian point

【现行译法】 river-jing points; acupoint/acupuncture point/point; meridian point; Meridian Points; classical point; river point; channel point; acupoint; jing (river) points; the jing (river) points; meridian acupoint

【推荐译法】 1) meridian points; 2) *jing* (river) points

【翻译说明】 经穴有两种不同的含义，或指经穴总称，或指五输穴中的经穴。根据上下文语境，可译为 meridian points 或 *jing* (river) points。

引例 Citations:

◎ 今于逐脉之下，载其经穴，与其病证，兼及浮络、经筋之病，共为一编。(《圣济总录·经脉统论》卷一百九十一)

（现在于每个经脉之下，记载经脉腧穴与主治的病证，同时论及浮络、经筋的病证，共编为本书的一部分。）

The acupoints of each meridian and their indications, together with the corresponding diseases and patterns of floating collaterals and meridian sinews, are now recorded in one section. (*Comprehensive Recording of Divine Assistance*)

◎ 有浮肿者，不可治络，宜疗经穴也。(《太素·咳论》)

（对于面部浮肿等症，不可针刺络脉，而应针刺有关经脉五输穴中的经穴。）

For facial edema and other diseases, the collaterals should not be punctured. Instead, acupuncture should be applied at the *jing* (river) points (one type of the five transport points) of the relevant meridians. (*Grand Simplicity*) qíxué

# 奇穴

Extra Points

奇穴，又称经外奇穴、经外穴，指十二经脉与督脉、任脉以外的腧穴。虽未归入十四经穴的范围，但却是有具体位置和名称的经验效穴。杨继洲《针灸大成》卷三"穴有奇正策"解释说："自正穴之外，又益之以奇穴焉……夫有针灸，则必有会数法之全，有数法则必有所定之穴，而奇穴者，则又旁通于正穴之外，以随时疗症者也。"

The term refers to the acupoints located beyond those on the fourteen meridians (the twelve meridians, the governor vessel, and the conception vessel). Although they are not included in the fourteen meridian points, the extra points have their specific locations, names, and therapeutic effects based on clinical experiences. Yang Jizhou explained in Volume 3 of *The Great Compendium of Acupuncture and Moxibustion*: "There are also some extra points besides the regular points… For acupuncture and moxibustion, there must be a set of numbers and rules. The numbers and rules specify the acupoints. The extra points are supplementary to the regular acupoints, and can be used to treat various diseases at any time."

【曾经译法】 extra-point; extra points

【现行译法】 extraordinary points/extra-meridian-points/off-meridian points; extraordinary acupoints/extra acupoints; meridian points/river points; Extra Points; extra point; extra acupoint; meridian/channel points

【推荐译法】 extra points

【翻译说明】 针灸经络和穴位术语的翻译目前已经非常规范，遵循世界卫生组织总部针灸穴名国际标准化科学组会议审定通过的《标准针灸穴名》，将"奇穴"翻译成 extra points。

引例 Citations:

◎ 若是腹痛兼闭结，支沟奇穴保平安。（《扁鹊神应针灸玉龙经·一百二十穴玉龙歌》）

　　（若患者腹痛兼有闭结不通，针刺奇穴支沟可保平安。）

If the patient has abdominal pain and stagnation, needling *zhigou* (SJ6), one of the extra points, can restore health. (*Bianque's Miraculous Yulong Classic of Acupuncture and Moxibustion*)

◎ 圣人取穴，三百六十有六，按岁之三百六十六日也。后人以为未尽，更取奇穴，是犹置闰月也。（《针灸问对》卷上）

　　（高明的医生取穴有三百六十六个腧穴，乃是参照一年有三百六十六天。后人认为没有穷尽，更取奇穴，这好像设置闰月。）

For a sage, there are 366 acupoints, corresponding to 366 days in a year. Practitioners in later generations believed that there should be more and found the extra points, which is like the setting of the leap month. (*Catechism on Acupuncture and Moxibustion*) luòxué

# 络穴

*Luo* (Connecting) Points

　　络穴，是位于十五络脉起始处的一类腧穴，本为十五络脉名称，后来演变为络穴名称，即十二经脉之别，督、任脉之别以及脾之大络，分别名为列缺、通里、内关、支正、偏历、外关、飞扬、丰隆、光明、公孙、大钟、蠡沟、会阴、长强、大包。络穴主病多是所属经脉病候及该络脉本身循行所过处病症。

The term refers to a group of acupoints located at the beginning of the fifteen collaterals. The name of *luo* (connecting) points is derived from the fifteen collaterals, i.e., the collaterals of the twelve meridians, the governor vessel, the conception vessel, and the great collateral vessel of the spleen. *Luo* (connecting) points include *lieque* (LU7), *tongli* (HT4), *neiguan* (PC6), *zhizheng* (SI7), *pianli* (LI6), *waiguan* (SJ5), *feiyang* (BL58), *fenglong* (ST39), *guangming* (GB37), *gongsun* (SP4), *dazhong* (KI4), *ligou* (LR5), *huiyin* (CV1), *changqiang* (GV1), and *dabao* (SP21). They are mostly used to treat the diseases and patterns that belong to the corresponding meridians and collaterals.

【曾经译法】 collateral point; luo points (acupuncture points of the collateral channels); collateral points; network point [new]; connecting point [old]

【现行译法】 collateral acupoints; connecting point; Connecting Points; Luo-Connecting Point; Luo-(connecting) point; luo points; collateral vessel; Luo-connecting acupoint; collateral acupoint

【推荐译法】 *luo* (connecting) points

【翻译说明】 既往译法中，基本都采用 connecting 来翻译"络"，建议加上拼音，能够凸显中医特色腧穴的概念。

引例 Citations:

◎ 一十二经，每经络各有一络穴，外有三络穴……此一十五络穴之辨也。
（《针经指南·络说》）

> （十二经脉，每条经脉各有一个络穴，另外有三个络穴……这是
> 十五络穴的判别。）

Each of the twelve meridians has a *luo* (connecting) point. Besides, there are another three... This is how to identify the fifteen *luo* (connecting) points. (*Guide to Acupuncture Classic*)

◎ 手阳明大肠经病，可刺本经表之原穴，即合谷穴也，复刺肺经里之络穴，即列缺穴也。（《医宗金鉴·刺灸心法要诀》）

> （手阳明大肠经的病证，可刺本经属表的原穴，即合谷穴；再刺
> 肺经属里的络穴，即列缺穴。）

To treat diseases in the Large Intestine Meridian of Hand-*yangming*, *hegu* (LI4), the original acupoint of this meridian, which belongs to the exterior, can be needled first, and then *lieque* (LU6), the *luo* (connecting) point of the lung meridian, which belongs to the interior, can be needled. (*Golden Mirror of the Medical Tradition*) jīngqì

# 经气

Meridian Qi

经气，也称为脉气、经脉之气，指分布运行于经脉的气。经脉通过经气的运行，调节全身各部的功能，协调阴阳，从而使整个机体保持协调和阴阳动态平衡。经气反映着人体的功能状态，针灸亦是通过调节经气达到治疗目的，故针刺过程中，刺法、行针和补泻手法均注重经气。

The term refers to the qi that circulates and is distributed in the meridians. The meridians regulate all parts of the body and coordinate yin and yang through the movement of meridian qi to maintain harmony, the dynamic balance of yin and yang, in the whole body. As meridian qi reflects the functional state of the human body, it can be regulated by acupuncture to treat diseases. Therefore, in the process of acupuncture, needling methods as well as reinforcing and reducing techniques are emphasized to regulate meridian qi.

【曾经译法】 vital energy circulating in the channels/healthy energy; the qi (vital energy) of the channels (the channel qi); channel-energy; channel qi; meridian qi

【现行译法】 meridian qi; Channel-qi; Meridian Qi; channel Qi; channel qi; the qi of the channels (the channel qi); meridian essence

【推荐译法】 meridian qi

【翻译说明】 "经气"即"经脉之气"的简称。经脉的标准译法为 meridian，可做定语，组成 meridian qi，使译文简明、准确。

引例 Citations:

◎ 脉气流经，经气归于肺，肺朝百脉，输精于皮毛。(《素问·经脉别论》)

    (经脉之气流行于经脉之中，上达于肺，肺又将经脉之气输送到全身经脉，直至皮毛。)

Meridian qi flows in the meridians, traveling up to the lung. The lung transports meridian qi to all meridians and vessels of the human body and distributes it at the skin and body hair. (*Plain Conversation*)

◎ 刺虚者须其实，刺实者须其虚，经气已至，慎守勿失。(《素问·宝命全形论》)

    (针刺虚证须用补法，针刺实证须用泻法，经脉之气已经到了，应慎重掌握，不失时机。)

In terms of acupuncture techniques, reinforcing should be used for deficiency patterns and reducing should be used for excess patterns. It is necessary to grasp the timing in the case of the arrival of meridian qi. (*Plain Conversation*) biāoběn

# 标本

Tip and Root

    标本，又称经脉标本，语出《灵枢·卫气》。标，树梢；本，树根。用以比喻十二经脉上下特定部位的关系和意义，四肢部为主为本，阳脉以头颈部、阴脉以背俞与腋胁为次为标。从经脉循行规律的角度而言，阳脉由四肢至头颈，故其本在四肢，其标在头颈部。阴脉由四肢循行至内脏，部分经脉循行至舌或腋，故其本在四肢，部分经脉的标在舌部或腋部；而背部亦有主治内脏病症的腧穴，故阴脉的标多在背部。

The term, also named the tip and root of meridians, originates from the "Defense Qi" of *Miraculous Pivot*. *Biao* means the tip or branch of a tree and *ben* means the root. *Biao Ben* (tip and root) describes the relationship and significance of the specific parts of the twelve meridians. The limbs are primary and considered as the root. The head and neck are secondary and considered as the tip for yang meridians, while the back, armpits, and ribs are the tip for yin meridians. From the perspective of meridian circulation, yang meridians run from the four limbs to the head and neck, so the limbs are considered as the "root," and the head and neck are considered as the "tip." Yin meridians run from the four limbs to the internal organs, some of which run to the tongue or armpits, so the limbs are considered as the "root," and the tongue or armpits are considered as the "tip" for some yin meridians. There are also acupoints for visceral diseases on the back of the human body, so the "tip" of yin meridians is mostly on the back.

【曾经译法】 the branch and the root (for a disease, it means the principal and the secondary aspects); biao (the secondary) and ben (the primary); branch and root; superficiality and origin, the incidental and the fundamental; the "branch" and the "root;" root and tip

【现行译法】 primary and secondary aspects/principle and subordinate aspects; branch and root; tip/incidental (标), root/the fundamental (本);

The incidental and the fundamental; superficiality and origin, incidental and fundamental; manifestation and root cause; symptom and root cause; the incidental and fundamental; biao (the secondary) and ben (the primary); treetop and root

【推荐译法】 tip and root

【翻译说明】 中医语境中，"标"常被译为 tip/manifestation/symptom，"本"常用 root/root cause 表示。单词 tip（尖端；树梢）和 root（根）能够比较形象地体现主次关系，也更简洁，建议把"标本"译为 tip and root。

引例 Citations:

◎ 能知六经标本者，可以无惑于天下。（《灵枢·卫气》）

（能够知道手足六经的标和本，在治疗复杂疾病时就能应对自如了。）

The knowledge of the "tip" and "root" in the six meridians of the hand and the foot enables one to address complex diseases with ease. (*Miraculous Pivot*)

◎ 盖以经脉所起之处为本，所出之处为标。（《灵枢集注》卷六）

（以经脉起始部位为本，出于体表部位为标。）

The starting position of a meridian is considered as the "root" while the corresponding part on the body surface is considered as the "tip." (*Collected Commentaries on the "Miraculous Pivot"*)

gēnjié

# 根结

Root and Knot

根结，指经脉的起始与结聚部位。语出《灵枢·卫气》。根，植物之根，引申为始、本原的意思；结，绳相连接，引申出聚、归结、终之义。用以比喻足六经上下特定部位间的内在关系，下肢远端部腧穴对头胸腹部具有特定治疗作用，即足经肢端腧穴的远隔效应。

The term refers to the starting and knotting portions of meridians. It originates from the "Defense Qi" of *Miraculous Pivot*. *Gen* (根) refers to the root of plants, whose figurative use is origin. *Jie* (结) means that the rope is connected, whose figurative use is gathering and ending. *Gen Jie* (root and knot) describes the internal relationship among specific parts of the six meridians of the foot. The acupoints at the distal part of the lower limbs have a specific therapeutic effect on the head, chest, and abdomen, that is, the distant effect of the acupoints at the extremities of the foot meridian.

【曾经译法】 root and knot; root and end (of meridians); root and knot/end

【现行译法】 gen and jie points; roots and endings of meridians; root and knot; starting and terminal points of meridian; starting and terminal point of meridian/channel; starting and terminal point; roots and knots

【推荐译法】 root and knot

【翻译说明】 "根"即"本"，与 root 对应。"结"指"结聚"，与 knot 对应。

引例 Citations:

◎ 不知根结，五脏六腑，折关败枢，开合而走，阴阳大失，不可复取。
（《灵枢·根结》）

> （不知道经脉的起始与结聚及五脏六腑的相互关系，就会导致六
> 经关守折损、枢纽败坏，以致开合不当，真气走泄，阴阳之气大
> 量损耗，针刺治疗也不能起作用了。）

If one does not know the root and knot and the interrelationships with the five *zang*-organs and the six *fu*-organs, it will cause damage to the pivoting of the six meridians, resulting in improper opening and closing, the leaking of genuine qi, and the significant loss of yin qi and yang qi. If so, acupuncture therapy will not work either. (*Miraculous Pivot*)

◎ 下者为根，上者为结。疾之中人，不可胜数，而治之者，当审根结之
本末。（《类经·经络类》）

> （经脉的下部为根，上部为结。邪气侵袭人体发病，不可胜数，
> 而治疗必须审察经脉的根结、标本。）

The lower part of the meridian is the root, and the upper part is the knot. There are countless cases of pathogenic factors attacking the human body, and the root and knot of meridians must be examined. (*Classified Classics*)

# 气街

Qi Pathway; *Qichong* (ST30)

气街，指经气聚集运行的通路。首见于《灵枢·卫气》："请言气街：胸气有街，腹气有街，头气有街，胫气有街。"说明头、胸、腹、胫部有经气聚集运行的通路。气街横贯脏腑经络，纵向分为头气街、胸气街、腹气街、胫气街。诊断上，气街可以反映病候，且多为脏腑之疾。如常用的胸腹切诊、俞募穴压诊等诊断方法均与气街理论有关。治疗上，俞募配穴、前后配穴、近部取穴等针灸配穴法，也均以气街理论为依据。此外，气街也是胃经经穴气冲穴的别名。

The term refers to a passage through which meridian qi accumulates and flows. It was first documented in the "Defense Qi" of *Miraculous Pivot*: "There are pathways for the converging and flow of meridian qi in the head, chest, abdomen, and shin." The qi pathway crosses the *zang-fu* organs, meridians, and collaterals, and is divided into four parts: the head qi pathway, the chest qi pathway, the abdominal qi pathway, and the tibial qi pathway. In terms of diagnosis, qi pathway can reflect the diseases and patterns, most of which are *zang-fu* diseases. The commonly used diagnostic methods such as palpation on the chest and abdomen and compression methods on *shu-mu* acupoints are all related to the theory of qi pathway. In terms of treatment, some methods of acupoint combination, such as *shu-mu* point combination, anterior-posterior point combination, selection of adjacent points, are also based on the theory of qi pathway. In addition, the term may also refer to *qichong* (ST30), an acupoint of the stomach meridian.

【曾经译法】 the area in the groin where pulsation of the femoral artery can be felt; pathway of qi; qi thoroughfare; ST-30 (Qi Thoroughfare); 1) tunnel of meridian qi, 2) Qi chong point, 3) qi passage

【现行译法】 qi passage/pathway of qi/qi thoroughfare; pathway of meridian

Qi, qi passageway; qijie; qi pathway; qi path

【推荐译法】 qi pathway; *qichong* (ST30)

【翻译说明】 根据释义，"街"指"通路"，故而"气街"译为 pathway 较妥。此外，气街是气冲穴的别名，为胃经经穴，可音译为 *qichong* (ST30)。

引例 Citations:

◎ 胸、腹、头、胻四种，身之要也。四处气行之道，谓之街也。(《太素》卷十)

（胸、腹、头、胫四个部位，为身体的要冲。四处气行的道路，称为"气街"。）

The chest, abdomen, head, and shin are the important parts of the human body. The passages where qi runs in the aforementioned four parts are called qi pathways. (*Grand Simplicity*)

◎ 此四街者，乃胸、腹、头、胫之气，所聚所行之道路，故谓之气街。(《类经·经络类》)

（这四街即胸、腹、头、胫之气汇聚、运行的道路，因此称为"气街"。）

The four passages, through which the qi of the chest, abdomen, head, and shin converges and runs, are called "qi pathways." (*Classified Classics*) déqì

# 得气

*Deqi* Sensation

　　得气是指针刺入腧穴后，通过使用提插、捻转、循法、刮法等手法，使针刺部位的腧穴产生特殊的感觉和反应。也称针感、气至。得气时医者的刺手能体会到针下沉紧、涩滞或针体颤动等反应；患者感觉针刺部位有酸、麻、胀、重等反应，或有酸麻、酸胀、麻胀、酸痛等复合感觉，有些穴位还会出现热、凉、痒、蚁行、流动、触电等感觉，这类感觉也可能沿着一定方向和部位传导或扩散。得气是施行针刺产生治疗作用、针刺取得疗效的关键，也是正确定穴，选择行针、补泻手法和判定患者经气盛衰、针刺效应、疾病预后的依据，是针刺过程中进一步实施手法的基础。

The term describes the special feeling and sensation of the acupoints after the needle is inserted into the acupoint with lifting-thrusting, twirling, massage along the meridians, scraping, and other methods. It is also known as needling sensation or qi arrival. When qi is felt, the acupuncturist can feel the needle sinking, rough or shaking. The patient can feel soreness, numbness, distention, and heaviness at the acupuncture site, or there are combined sensations such as soreness and numbness, soreness and distention, numbness and distention, and soreness and pain. There will also be sensations of heat, cold, itching, ant moving, flowing, and electric shock. Such feelings may be transmitted or diffused along a certain direction. *Deqi* sensation is the key to the therapeutic effect of acupuncture. It is also the basis for the correct selection of acupoints, the selection of needling methods, the manipulation of reinforcing and reducing techniques, and the determination of the relative predominance of a patient's meridian qi, the acupuncture effect, and the prognosis of the disease. Besides, it is the basis for further needling manipulations.

【曾经译法】 normal sensation felt by the patient and doctor during acupuncture; deqi (needling sensations); getting the acupuncture feeling; getting qi, arrival of qi; obtain qi; obtaining qi; acu-esthesia

【现行译法】needling response/needling sensation/arrival of qi; getting the qi; Arrival of qi; getting sensation of acupuncture; obtaining qi; acuesthesia; arrival of qi in acupuncture; arrival of Qi

【推荐译法】*deqi* sensation

【翻译说明】译文 arrival of qi 偏于"气至"；obtaining qi 偏指针灸师的指下感觉。"得气"的含义包括患者和针灸师双方的感觉。目前学术期刊论文均已约定俗成使用 *deqi*，建议"得气"翻译为 *deqi* sensation，突出感觉。


引例 Citations:


◎ 吸则内针，无令气忤，静以久留，无令邪布，吸则转针，以得气为故。（《素问·离合真邪论》）

> （吸气时进针，勿使气逆，要留针静候其气不让病邪扩散；吸气时捻针，以得气为目的。）

The patient is asked to breathe in when the needles are inserted to prevent reverse flow of qi and the needles are retained to prevent spread of pathogenic qi. The needles are rotated when the patient breathes in for the purpose of *deqi* sensation. (*Plain Conversation*)


◎ 言下针若得气来速，则病易痊，而效亦速也。气若来迟，则病难愈，而有不治之忧。（《针灸大成·标幽赋》）

> （说针刺后若得气迅速，病就容易治愈，取效也快。若得气迟缓，病就不容易治愈，而有不治的忧患。）

If *deqi* sensation is felt quickly after needling, it will be easy to cure the disease and quick effects can be obtained. If *deqi* sensation is felt slowly, it will be difficult to cure the disease, and there is a possibility that the disease is incurable. (*The Great Compendium of Acupuncture and Moxibustion*) shǒuqì

# 守气

Examine Qi; Keep Qi

守气，在《黄帝内经》中一指针刺前的诊查过程，通过脉诊体察把握患者的气血变化，与"守神""守机"内涵相近；二指针刺得气之后，通过一定操作来维持经气，使经气留守不去。后世多指后者，即强调在针刺得气后，慎守勿失，留守不去。具体操作也包括医患两个方面，就医者而言，得气时不要随便改变针刺方向和针刺深度，宜手不离针，持针不动，针尖不要偏离已得气之处。或用治神运气法，贯气于指，守气勿失；或用较轻柔平和手法，促使经气徐徐而至，绕于针下。就患者而言，要积极配合治疗，安神定志，意守感传。

The term refers to the process and techniques before acupuncture treatment. It has two meanings in *Huangdi's Inner Cannon of Medicine*. The first one refers to the process of examination before application of acupuncture, where the practitioner observes the changes of the patient's qi and blood through pulse diagnosis. It is similar to "keeping the spirit" (*shoushen*) and "examining the opportunity" (*shouji*). The second one, which is mostly used by later generations, refers to maintaining the meridian qi through certain manipulations after *deqi* sensation is experienced so that the meridian qi stays. The specific manipulations require cooperation between the practitioner and the patient. For the practitioner, he or she shall not change the direction or the depth of the needles when *deqi* sensation is obtained. It is advised to keep his or her hand on the needle, and make sure the needle located in situ after *deqi* sensation is felt. Besides, the method of governing the spirit and qi can also be used, where the practitioner guides qi to the fingers, and make it stay. The practitioner can also apply gentle manipulations to guide the meridian qi to come slowly and make it move around the needle. When it comes to the patient, he or she should be compliant (with the treatment), calm nerves and minds to maintain qi, and feel its movement.

【曾经译法】 maintaining needling sensation

【现行译法】 keeping the needling response; maintaining needling sensation; keeping qi

【推荐译法】 1) examine qi; 2) keep qi

【翻译说明】 "守气"有两层含义，一指通过脉诊体察把握患者的气血变化，可译为 examine qi；二指使经气留守不去，可译为 keep qi。


引例 Citations:


◎ 上守机者，知守气也……空中之机，清静以微者，针以得气，密意守气勿失也。(《灵枢·小针解》)

（上守机，是说高明的医生懂得把握气机变化的规律……空中之机，清静以微，是说针下已经得气，就要周密注意气的往来，不能失去针刺补泻的有利时机。）

The superb practitioners know how to seize the opportunity as they know how to examine the changes of qi... When *deqi* sensation is obtained, attention shall be paid to the flow of qi to grasp the opportunity for reinforcing or reducing through needling manipulations. (*Miraculous Pivot*)

◎ 寒清者，内因之虚寒，宜深取之，静以守气，故如人不欲行也。(《灵枢集注》卷一)

（寒凉的病证，因内有虚寒，应深刺，静候守气，好像人不想行走。）

For cold patterns, the needle shall be deeply inserted due to internal accumulation of deficient cold. The practitioner shall wait and keep qi just like a person is reluctant to leave. (*Collected Commentaries on "Miraculous Pivot"*)

shǒushén

# 守神

Keep the Spirit

　　守神，本义指观察、把握人体气血之微妙变化。后世引申指医者在进针后所持的专心态度，以及针刺得气后患者聚精会神、体会针感的留针过程。具体包含以下两个方面：一、进针后着意守神。进针后，医者守神则静候气至，仔细体察针下指感以辨气，合理调整针刺的深浅和方向；患者守神则可促使针下得气，令气易行。二、行针宜移神制神而守神。针刺入一定深度后，医者宜采用各种催气手法，促使针下得气。同时又须观察患者的神态和目光，通过医患之间的目光交接，使患者神情安定。

The term originally refers to observing and detecting the subtle changes of qi and blood of the human body. It has been used later to refer to the practitioner's attentiveness after needle insertion as well as the patient's concentration and acupuncture sensation in the process of needle retention after *deqi* sensation is experienced. Specifically, it includes the following two aspects. First, both the practitioner and the patient keep the spirit carefully after needle insertion. For the practitioner, he or she shall wait for qi to arrive and carefully observe the feeling under the finger to properly adjust the depth and direction of the needle; when the patient keeps the spirit, qi movement is easier and *deqi* sensation is promoted. Second, the practitioner should keep the spirit while moving and controlling the needling manipulation. After the needle reaches a certain depth, the practitioner shall apply various techniques to promote *deqi* sensation. At the same time, it is necessary for the practitioner to observe the patient and maintain eye contact to soothe and calm the patient.

【曾经译法】 spiritual concentration, full attention

【现行译法】 hold the spirit

【推荐译法】 keep the spirit

【翻译说明】 "守神"中的"神"为广义之精神，建议译为 spirit。基于类似术语结构翻译的一致性，可将"守神"译为 keep the spirit，同时也可根据上下文语境，灵活翻译"守神"。

引例 Citations:

◎ 小针之要，易陈而难入，粗守形，上守神。(《灵枢·九针十二原》)

（小针的关键所在，说起来容易，可是达到精微的境界却很难啊！粗工拘守形体，仅知在病位上针刺，高明的医工却懂得根据患者的神气变化针治疾病。）

For the crux of needling, it is easier said, yet it is difficult to reach the acme of perfection. The mediocre practitioners see nothing beyond the physical body and only apply acupuncture on the site of disease, whereas the superb practitioners know how to treat the disease according to the changes of the patient's spirit and qi. (*Miraculous Pivot*)

◎ 上守神者，守人之血气有余不足，可补泻也。(《灵枢·小针解》)

（上守神，就是指高明的医生，能够掌握患者的血气虚实，考虑是用补法还是泻法。）

The superb practitioners are able to detect the deficiency or excess of the patient's blood and qi, and use the method of reinforcement or reduction accordingly. (*Miraculous Pivot*) shǒujī

# 守机

Examine the Opportunity; Seize the Opportunity

守机，是以弓弩之机比喻守气之机，即观察脉气之虚实动静变化，掌握针刺的时机。"机"是事物运动变化的先兆、关键点，上工当把握住"机"，决不放过治疗的最佳时机。守机察"气至之动静"，守神察"血气有余不足"，均要依靠脉诊，守神与守机通过脉诊的联系而密切相关。脉诊的过程就是一个探求神机、体会气之逆顺出入的过程，守神与守机，就是要通过脉诊来把握气血的微妙变化与针刺治疗稍纵即逝的时机。

The term refers to observing the dynamic changes of deficiency and excess of pulse qi for applying needling appropriately. It uses the moment of shooting bows or crossbows as a metaphor for the sense of timing, which refers to the awareness of signs and the crucial point of changes. The superb practitioners will seize the best opportunity for treatment. The two processes, i.e., examining the opportunity to observe the dynamic changes of qi and keeping the spirit to detect the deficiency or excess of blood and qi, are to be completed via pulse diagnosis and so they are closely related. Pulse diagnosis is a process of exploring the spirit and timing to feel qi movement. It is the means that the practitioners understand the subtle changes of qi and blood in the processes of examining the opportunity and keeping the spirit so that they can seize the transient opportunity for acupuncture treatment.

【曾经译法】无

【现行译法】无

【推荐译法】1) examine the opportunity; 2) seize the opportunity

【翻译说明】本术语中的"机"即"变化之机"，既有"时机"，也有"枢机"的含义。守机既包括观察动态变化，发现变化之机，也包括及时抓住时机，给予治疗。根据上下文语境，可将"守机"译为 examine the opportunity 或 seize the opportunity。

引例 Citations:

◎ 刺之微在速迟，粗守关，上守机，机之动，不离其空。(《灵枢·九针十二原》)

　　(针刺的巧妙，在于如何运用疾徐手法。粗工拘守四肢关节的穴位治疗，高明的医生却能观察经气的变化。经气的循行，离不开腧穴。)

The subtlety of acupuncture lies in how to use the quick-slow technique. The mediocre practitioners are limited to the routine treatment of needling, whereas the superb practitioners can seize the opportunity to observe qi which circulates and infuses into acupoints. (*Miraculous Pivot*)

◎ 上守机者，知守气也。机之动不离其空者，知气之虚实，用针之徐疾也。(《灵枢·小针解》)

　　(上守机，是说高明的医生懂得把握气机变化的规律。机之动不离其空，是说只有了解腧穴中气的虚实变化，才能运用疾徐补泻手法。)

The superb practitioners know how to seize the opportunity as they know how to detect the changes of qi. Only when they know the changes of qi deficiency and excess in acupoints can they properly apply the quick-slow technique of reinforcement and reduction. (*Miraculous Pivot*) hòuqì

# 候气

Await Qi

候气，指测候、等候、把握气的变化而针刺的方法。这里的"气"包括自然之气和人体之气，要求根据气的盛衰和运行时间节律进行针刺，具体涉及依据人体经气运行把握针刺时机，以及依据天时（四时寒暑、月相盈亏等）而针刺。后世扩大了候气的外延，包括了望色诊脉等判断气血状况的诊察方法，把握患者针刺反应的方法及某些具体针刺操作，并发展出子午流注针法。如对于气血虚弱或久病年迈的患者，有时针刺得气较慢或难以得气，可将刺入的针留在穴位内，或对其间歇施以提插、捻转等手法，进行运针，使之气至。其中留针而等待气至者，为静留针候气；留针后间歇进行运针以等待气至者，为动留针候气。

The term refers to the needling methods based on assessing, awaiting, and grasping the changes of qi, including the qi of nature and human body. Acupuncture is expected to be applied based on the waxing and waning of qi and the temporal rhythm of qi movement. Specifically, the timing of acupuncture is determined according to the movement of meridian qi in the human body and natural changes (e.g., four seasons and moon phases). Later generations expand the connotation of awaiting qi. It includes the diagnostic methods such as inspection of the complexion and pulse diagnosis for determining the state of qi and blood, the method of observing the patient's reaction towards acupuncture, and some specific needling techniques such as midnight-midday ebb flow acupuncture. For example, for patients with deficiency of qi and blood and those with prolonged disease or in an old age, *deqi* sensation might appear more slowly or with difficulty. In these cases, the practitioner can leave needles in situ, or use lifting-thrusting technique and twisting-twirling technique intermittently to facilitate the arrival of qi. Therefore, awaiting qi in needle retention can be divided into the dynamic type (intermittent needling techniques applied) and the static type (no needling techniques applied).

【曾经译法】 wait for the normal sensation during acupuncture treatment; waiting for qi; wait for the coming of normal sensation during acupuncture treatment; awaiting qi; waiting for qi arrival

【现行译法】 waiting for arrival of qi/waiting for suitable time for treatment; waiting normal sensation in acupuncture treatment/waiting for acupuncture sensation; Waiting for Qi; waiting for Qi after needling; waiting for qi arrival; awaiting qi; waiting for mild tingling or aching sensation in acupuncture; waiting for Qi arrival

【推荐译法】 await qi

【翻译说明】 按照简洁性的原则，建议将"候气"译为 await qi；其含义的具体内容可以根据上下文进行诠释和理解。


引例 Citations:


◎ 谨候气之所在而刺之，是谓逢时。病在于三阳，必候其气在于阳而刺之；病在于三阴，必候其气在阴分而刺之。(《灵枢·卫气行》)

（谨慎地候察气所在部位而及时针刺的，叫做逢时。病在三阳经的，一定候其气在阳分的时候针刺；病在三阴经的，一定候其气在阴分的时候针刺。）

The perfect timing for applying acupuncture is based on careful observation of the location of qi. If the disease is located in the three yang meridians, acupuncture shall be applied when qi is in the yang section; if the disease is in the three yin meridians, acupuncture shall be applied when qi is in the yin section. (*Miraculous Pivot*)


◎ 用针之法，以候气为先。(《针灸大成》卷四)

（针刺治疗疾病的大法，以候气为先导。）

Acupuncture treatment prioritizes awaiting qi. (*The Great Compendium of Acupuncture and Moxibustion*)

# 调气

Regulate Qi

调气，指通过对机体失常之气的调节，使其恢复调和状态。气机正常是维持全身生理功能正常的基础，而机体气机失调，即脏腑气机升降出入功能失常就会产生各种疾病。因此，调理气机是治疗疾病的重要法则。针灸治疗疾病就是通过采用各种刺灸方法，应用补虚泻实等手法，刺激腧穴，以激发经气，调理气机，使脏腑气血、阴阳趋于平衡，从而使疾病得以痊愈。故《类经·针刺类》言："调气者，察其虚实往来而调和之也。"《素问·至真要大论》将调气的概念从针灸之补泻，发展为中医诸多治法，使调气概念扩展到整个中医治法范畴之中。

The term refers to the process of adjusting abnormal qi of the body to restore harmony. Normal qi movement is the basis for maintaining normal physiological function of the whole body, whereas disorder of qi movement, that is, disorder of the ascending and descending of qi in *zang-fu* organs, will cause various diseases. Therefore, regulating qi is an important principle for treating diseases. Acupuncture and moxibustion work through various methods that stimulate acupoints, such as reinforcing deficiency and reducing excess, to activate meridian qi and regulate qi movement, which will restore balance of qi and blood as well as yin and yang in *zang-fu* organs. In this way the disease can be cured. Therefore, *Classified Classics* states: "Regulating qi means observing the dynamic changes of deficiency and excess to restore balance in the human body." Additionally, *Plain Conversation* has developed the concept of regulating qi from reinforcing and reducing in acupuncture and moxibustion to many other therapeutic methods so that regulating qi applies to the whole treatment category of traditional Chinese medicine.

【曾经译法】 regulate the vital energy; promoting the flow of qi; regulating qi; regulate qi; regulating respiration

【现行译法】regulating qi; regulating breath; Regulate qi; Regulating Qi Flow; Qi regulation; adjusting qi; promoting the flow of qi

【推荐译法】regulate qi

【翻译说明】调，即调理，既往译法中主要使用的动词包括 regulate, adjust 和 promote。从"调理"的含义看，regulate 较妥。

引例 Citations:

◎ 是故工之用针也，知气之所在，而守其门户。明于调气，补泻所在，徐疾之意，所取之处。(《灵枢·官能》)

（所以医生用针，应该知道脉气的运行所在，选取相应的腧穴治疗。明白如何调气，什么应补，什么应泻，进针或快或慢，该取什么穴位。）

The practitioners who apply acupuncture shall be aware of the circulation of pulse qi and choose corresponding acupoints. They shall learn how to regulate qi, when to use reinforcing method, when to use reducing method, whether the needle should be inserted quickly or slowly, and what acupoints should be taken. (*Miraculous Pivot*)

◎ 调气之方，必别阴阳，定其中外，各守其乡，内者内治，外者外治，微者调之，其次平之，盛者夺之，汗之下之，寒热温凉，衰之以属，随其攸利。(《素问·至真要大论》)

（调气治病的方法，必须分别阴阳，确定在内在外，各依其病之所在，在内的治其内，在外的治其外，病轻的调理，较重的平治，病势盛的就攻夺，或用汗法，或用下法，要分辨病邪的寒、热、温、凉，根据病气的病位、病性使之消退，要随其所宜。）

In terms of regulating qi to treat diseases, the practitioners must differentiate yin and yang, determine the internal or external location of diseases, and choose countermeasures accordingly. For mild cases, regulate the body; for severe cases, treat the disease in a neutral way. When the disease attacks with great momentum, drastic therapeutic methods such as sweating or purging can be used. The nature of pathogenic qi (i.e., cold, hot, warm, and cool) shall be analyzed, and disease location shall be identified before treatment is applied to remove diseases. (*Plain Conversation*) zhēnbiān

# 针砭

Acupuncture; Point out the Mistakes

针砭，古代一种以石针刺经脉穴道的治疗方法，后比喻发现和指正错误，力求改正。砭，即石针，中国最古老的医疗用具，后改用金属为针治病。

The term originally refers to a therapeutic method in ancient China that stimulates meridians and acupoints with stone needles. Later it is used as a metaphor for discovering and pointing out the mistakes for correction. *Bian*, namely stone needle, is the oldest form of medical appliance in China, which was later replaced by metal needle.

【曾经译法】 无

【现行译法】 无

【推荐译法】 1) acupuncture; 2) point out the mistakes

【翻译说明】 根据上下文不同语境，可翻译为 1) acupuncture; 2) point out the mistakes。

引例 Citation:

◎ 陇州道士曾若虚者，善医，尤得针砭之妙术。(《西斋话记》)

（陇州道士曾若虚，擅长医术，尤其掌握针刺治疗的妙术。）

Zeng Ruoxu, a Daoist from Longzhou (the present Longxian County in the Shaanxi Province), was good at treating diseases, especially with acupuncture therapy. (*Stories from Xizhai*) yàodàobìngchú

# 药到病除

The Disease Is Cured as Soon as Medicine Is Taken.

药到病除，即药一经服用，疾病就根除了。形容医术高明，药物灵验。也比喻措施、办法十分有效，问题迅速得到解决。

The term refers to the good efficacy of a medicine, meaning that the disease is eliminated as soon as the medicine is taken. It is used to describe the practitioner's excellent medical skills and that his or her prescription takes effect quickly. It also means that measures are very effective and problems are thus solved quickly.

【曾经译法】无

【现行译法】无

【推荐译法】The disease is cured as soon as medicine is taken.

【翻译说明】实际翻译中，常常需要根据上下文的具体情况，灵活翻译
　　　　　　"药到病除"。

引例 Citations:

◎ 药到病除，效如桴鼓。（《医学衷中参西录》）

　　（一经服药，疾病就根除了，疗效犹如鼓槌击鼓响应迅速。）

As soon as the medicine is taken, the disease is cured. The efficacy is instant, just like drum responding to the striking of drumsticks. (*Records of Chinese Medicine with Reference to Western Medicine*)

◎ 既然是对症下药，自然会药到病除。（《老生常谈·立竿见影》）

（既然是根据具体病证处方用药，自然用药后疾病就能根除。）

Since the medicine is prescribed according to the specific disease pattern, it will take effect instantly after administration. (*A Commonplace Talk of an Old Scholar*) yàoshízhīyán

# 药石之言

Good Advice Is like Medicine.

药石之言，指给人治病的良言，喻指规劝别人改过的良言。石，用以砭刺治病的石针。

The term refers to the good advice given to patients to help cure diseases. Figuratively, it means the good advice offered to persuade people to correct their mistakes. *Shi* (石, stone) refers to the stone needle used to cure diseases.

【曾经译法】无

【现行译法】无

【推荐译法】Good advice is like medicine.

【翻译说明】汉语中有"良药苦口""忠言逆耳"的类似说法。"药石之言"是借用良药的苦和针刺的痛，来比拟忠言不合心意。翻译可以简化处理。

引例 Citations:

◎（季辅）又上疏切谏时政得失，（太宗）特赐钟乳一剂，曰："进药石之言，故以药石相报"。（《旧唐书·高季辅传》）

（季辅又向太宗进呈奏章直言极谏时政的得失，太宗特赐钟乳一剂说："进谏药石一样的言论，因此以药石相回报。"）

Gao Jifu once again presented a memorial to Emperor Taizong to state the pros and cons of the current policy. Emperor Taizong specially granted him with a dose of *Zhongru* (*Stalactitum,* stalactite) and said, "What you wrote is like medicine, so I give you medicine as an award." (*History of the Early Tang Dynasty*)

◎ 财物过多耗人精血，损人寿命，此亦药石之言。(《聊斋志异》)

（财物过多就会耗损人的精血，折损人的寿命，这也是规劝人改过的良言。）

Excessive property will consume people's essence and blood, and thus shorten their lifespan. This is also a piece of good advice like medicine. (*Strange Tales from Make-do Studio*) gāndǎn-xiāngzhào

# 肝胆相照

Show Utter Devotion to Each Other

肝胆相照，即肝与胆关系密切，互相照应。中医学认为肝与胆经脉相互络属，同主疏泄，共同发挥协助消化的作用；而且肝为将军之官，主谋虑，胆为中正之官，主决断，肝胆相互配合，则人的思维正常，遇事果断。肝胆之间关系密切，后以此形容亲密的关系，以及坦诚交往共事，相互照应。

The term refers to the close relationship between the liver and the gallbladder. Traditional Chinese medicine believes that the liver and the gallbladder are connected with each other through meridians and collaterals, and they govern free flow of qi and assist digestion together. Moreover, the liver functions like a general, devising strategies; the gallbladder functions like a justice officer, controlling decision-making. They coordinate with each other and serve for a person's normal thinking and decision-making abilities. The relationship between the liver and the gallbladder is intimate. The term is also used to describe the intimacy between people who are sincere with each other and show care for each other.

【曾经译法】无

【现行译法】无

【推荐译法】show utter devotion to each other

【翻译说明】本词条来源于中医对肝胆关系的认识，翻译时可采取"意译"方法，把深层的含义表达出来，可译为 show utter devotion to each other。

引例 Citations:

◎ 所恃知己，肝胆相照，临书不惮倾倒。(《与陈察院文龙书》)

　　(我所依靠的是知己的人，能真心相待，在写信的时候不怕使用
　　倾慕的文字。)

Whom I rely on are those who know me and we can show utter devotion to each other, so I am not afraid of using admiring words in letters. (*A Letter to Chen Wenlong*)

◎ 肝胆相照，斯为腹心之友。(《幼学琼林》卷二)

　　(坦诚相见，可以畅所欲言，才是推心置腹的朋友。)

True friends are those who can show utter devotion to each other and are able to express their opinions freely. (*Children's Enlightenment Reading Materials*) qìnrénxīnpí

# 沁人心脾

Gladden the Heart and Refresh the Mind

沁人心脾，即芳香的气味渗入了心和脾，常用来形容芳香凉爽的空气或饮料使人感到舒适。也形容诗歌和文章优美动人，给人清新爽朗的感觉。

The term, literally meaning fragrance permeating the heart and the spleen, is often used to describe the fragrant, cool air or drinks that are refreshing and comforting. It can also be used to describe the elegance of poems and articles that give people a feeling of refreshment.

【曾经译法】无

【现行译法】无

【推荐译法】gladden the heart and refresh the mind

【翻译说明】"沁人心脾"来源于中医对心脾功能的认识。心藏神，脾藏意。因此本词条借用了中医的心脾概念，用以表达"让人感受深刻""感人肺腑"之意。翻译时可视具体语境进行意译。

引例 Citations:

◎ 刑书蔚州魏公环溪一诗，极令人感动……予谓五六句最沁人心脾。（《带经堂诗话》卷首）

（刑部尚书蔚州魏环溪一诗，极令人感动……我认为有五六句最感人肺腑。）

A poem written by Wei Huanxi, a native of Yuzhou (the present Yuxian County in Hebei Province) and the Minister of Penalty, is very touching. There are five or six lines affecting me deeply. (*Remarks on Poetry in Daijingtang*)

◎ 坦易者，多触景生情，因事起意，眼前景，口头语，自能沁人心脾，耐人咀嚼。(《瓯北诗话》卷四)

> (浅显易懂的诗，大多是因为看见眼前的景象而引发内心种种情绪，或是因为事件而兴起的意念，描写的是眼前景，使用的是口头语，读起来让人感受深刻，意味深长，值得再三玩味。)

Easy-to-understand poems are usually written when the author is inspired by what he sees or by an event, whence various emotions or thoughts arise. The scene is described in plain language, yet the words affect the readers deeply and are worth pondering over. (*Remarks on Poetry by Zhao Yi*) xīnpíng-qìhé

# 心平气和

## Peace of Mind and Harmony of Qi

心平气和，指思想或精神平静没有不安或压抑的感情。人在情绪平稳、平静，不是起伏跌宕的时候，气血运行会处在最和谐的状态，也就是最健康的状态。相反，情绪剧烈波动，就会打乱这个平衡、协调的状态，而导致疾病的发生。如《素问·举痛论》说："余知百病生于气也，怒则气上，喜则气缓，悲则气消，恐则气下，寒则气收，炅则气泄，惊则气乱，劳则气耗，思则气结。"

The term refers to the peace of mind or serenity of spirit free from anxiety and depression. When a person is in a stable and calm mood without swings, he or she will be in the healthiest state where qi and blood movement is the most harmonious. On the contrary, drastic mood swings would disrupt such a balanced and coordinated state and further lead to the occurrence of diseases. For example, *Plain Conversation* states that "I understand that all diseases are caused by qi disorders: rage drives qi upward; excessive joy slackens qi; excessive sorrow exhausts qi; excessive fear causes qi sinking; excessive cold causes qi to contract; excessive heat causes discharge of qi; excessive fright deranges qi; over-exertion consumes qi; and over-thinking binds qi."

【曾经译法】 无

【现行译法】 无

【推荐译法】 peace of mind and harmony of qi

【翻译说明】 "心平气和"是常用四字成语，其译文通常会根据具体语境灵活调整。中医学认为，心主神志，心平则气和，建议译为 peace of mind and harmony of qi。

引例 Citations:

◎ 心平气和是一药，不忌人美是一药。(《遵生八笺》卷二)

　　(心绪平静、气血调和是一种药，不嫉妒他人之美也是一种药。)

Peace of mind and harmony of qi are like medicines, so is being not jealous of others. (*Eight-section Book on Health Preservation*)

◎ 犯此症者，养气凝神，静坐忘言，心平气和者，十中曾愈二三人而已。(《银海精微补》卷三)

　　(罹患这种病症，养气凝神，静坐忘言，心平气和的，十个人中
　　曾有两三个人病愈而已。)

For those who suffer from this disease, if they are able to nourish qi, concentrate their attention, and meditate in silence with the peace of mind and harmony of qi, two or three out of ten patients will restore health. (*A Supplement to Essentials of the Silver Sea*) miàoshǒu-huíchūn

# 妙手回春

Bring the Dying Back to Life

妙手回春，颂扬医师的医术高明，能治好重病。妙手，高妙的技术。回春，使春天重返，比喻将快死的人救活。

The term is used to praise doctors for their superb expertise and ability to effect a miraculous cure and bring the dying back to life. *Miaoshou* (妙手) means ingenious skills; *huichun* (回春), literally bringing back the spring, is a metaphor for saving the dying.

【曾经译法】无

【现行译法】无

【推荐译法】bring the dying back to life

【翻译说明】"妙手回春"是常用四字成语，通过比喻修辞，赞扬医生的高明医术。"回春"即"起死回生"，建议译为 bring the dying back to life。

引例 Citations:

◎ 天彪、希真齐声道："全仗先生妙手回春。"（《荡寇志》第四十四回）

Tianbiao and Xizhen said in chorus, "It's all up to your excellent medical skills that bring the dying back to life." (*The Sequel of All Men Are Brothers*)

◎ 什么"妙手回春"，什么"是乃仁术"，匾上的字句，一时也记不清楚。（《官场现形记》第二十回）

I have a faint memory of the phrases on the inscribed tablet, something like "Bring the Dying Back to Life" and "This Embodies the Benevolence." (*Officialdom's True Features*) jú|ǐng quánxiāng

# 橘井泉香

Fragrance of Tangerine Leaves and Well Water

橘井泉香，是传统中医药史上赞颂高超医术、高尚医德的著名典故，出自葛洪《神仙传·苏仙公传》。相传苏耽生来异于常人，能够预见未来发生的事情。苏耽在汉文帝的时候受天命为天仙，天上的仪仗队降落苏宅来迎接他，在临行前他拉着母亲的手说："明年天下将流行瘟疫，咱们家庭院中的井水和橘树能治疗瘟疫。患瘟疫的人，给他井水一升，橘叶一枚，吃下橘叶、喝下井水就能治愈。"第二年果然疫病流行，远近悉求其母治疗，都以得井水及橘叶而治愈。自此，即以"橘井泉香"为良药之典。

The term refers to a well-known anecdote about doctors with superb expertise and noble medical ethics in the history of traditional Chinese medicine. According to Ge Hong's *Legend of Immortals*, there was a person named Su Dan who was born ingenious and able to foresee what would happen in the future. He became a heavenly immortal during the reign of Emperor Wen of the Han Dynasty. When the guard of honor from the heaven came down to Su's house to receive him, he took his mother's hand and said, "There will be a plague next year. It can be cured by the well water and tangerine trees in our courtyard. Those victims of the plague can be cured after drinking one *sheng* (200 ml) of well water and eating a tangerine leaf." As things turned out, the following year saw the prevalence of an epidemic disease. Patients from near and far came to seek help from Su's mother and they were cured by well water and tangerine leaves. Since then, the term "fragrance of tangerine leaves and well water" has been used as the symbol of good medicine.

【曾经译法】无

【现行译法】无

【推荐译法】fragrance of tangerine leaves and well water

【翻译说明】基于典故，建议采用直译的方法翻译"橘井泉香"，译为 fragrance of tangerine leaves and well water。

引例 Citation:

◎ 橘井泉香随地涌，杏林春暖落花飞。（《母重光遗稿·为彭子高医士题三联》）

The fragrance of tangerine leaves and well water flow; the flowers of apricot trees fly in warm spring. (*Posthumous Manuscript of Mu Chongguang*) xìnglín-chūnnuǎn

# 杏林春暖

Apricot Trees in Warm Spring

　　杏林春暖，是我国传统中医药史上赞颂高超医术、高尚医德的著名典故，出自《太平广记》。相传三国时候，吴国医生董奉医术精湛，助人为乐。他为人看病，却不收任何报酬，要求重病愈者种杏五株，轻病愈者种杏一株。如此数年，杏树成林。董奉把收获的杏子全部都换成粮食，用来救济穷苦的百姓。为了感激董奉的德行，有人写了"杏林春暖"的条幅挂在他家门口。从此，许多中药店都挂上了"杏林春暖"的匾额，"杏林"也逐渐成了中医药行业的代名词。

The term refers to a well-known anecdote about doctors with superb expertise and noble medical ethics in the history of traditional Chinese medicine (TCM). According to *Extensive Records Compiled in the Taiping Years*, during the Three Kingdoms period there was an eminent TCM practitioner named Dong Feng in the Kingdom of Wu. He treated patients free of charge. Instead of a monetary payment, he asked those who had recovered from serious diseases to plant five apricot trees and those from mild diseases to plant one apricot tree. After some years, a forest of apricot trees appeared. Dong Feng then traded all the apricots for grains to help the poor. To honor Dong Feng's virtue, someone hung up an inscribed tablet of "Apricot Trees in Warm Spring" on the gate of his residence. Since then, many pharmacies have copied the phrase on their inscribed boards. Gradually, the expression "apricot trees" is used to refer to the entire TCM profession.

【曾经译法】无

【现行译法】apricot trees/venerable doctors with good skills

【推荐译法】apricot trees in warm spring

【翻译说明】在教育部和国家语言文字工作委员会主持的"中华思想文化术语工程"第九辑中，根据不同语境，"杏林"译为 apricot

trees 或 venerable doctors with good skills。此处"杏林"译为
apricot trees 较妥，可反映中医典故。

引例 Citation:

◎ 权藉刀圭广救世，杏林春暖艳阳天。(《医学衷中参西录·和徐韵英二十
感怀原韵》)

（权借医术广救世，杏林春暖艳阳天。）

Save all living creatures with medical skills, and apricot trees will blossom in
warmth and sunshine. (*Records of Chinese Medicine with Reference to Western
Medicine*)

# 术语表  List of Concepts

# 索引 Index
(按音序 In Chinese Alphabetical Order)

# 参考文献 References

1.　广州中医学院《汉英常用中医词汇》编写组. 汉英常用中医词汇. 广州：广东科技出版社. 1982

2.　帅学忠. 汉英双解常用中医名词术语. 长沙：湖南科技出版社. 1983

3.　欧明. 汉英中医辞典. 广州：广东科技出版社；香港：三联书店香港分店. 1986

4.　汉英、汉法、汉德、汉日、汉俄医学大词典编纂委员会. 汉英医学大词典. 北京：人民卫生出版社. 1987

5.　北京中医药大学. 汉英中医药学词典. 北京：中医古籍出版社. 1994

6.　Nigel Wiseman（魏逎杰）. 英汉汉英中医词典. 长沙：湖南科学技术出版社. 1995

7.　李照国. 汉英中医药大词典. 北京：世界图书出版公司. 1997

8.　原一祥. 汉英双解中医大辞典. 北京：人民卫生出版社. 1997

9.　史载祥. 简明汉英日中医药词典. 北京：人民卫生出版社. 1998

10.　翁心植、胡亚美. 英汉汉英医学分科词典. 北京：世界图书出版公司. 1998

11.　张奇文主编，孙衡山译. 实用汉英中医词典. 济南：山东科学技术出版社. 2001

12.　Nigel Wiseman & Feng Ye. *A Practical Dictionary of Chinese Medicine*. 北京：人民卫生出版社. 2002

13.　李照国. 简明汉英中医词典. 上海：上海科技出版社. 2002

14.　谢竹藩. 新编汉英中医药分类词典. 北京：外文出版社. 2002

15.　张廷模. 汉英双解中医小辞典. 北京：人民卫生出版社. 2003

16.　左言富. 新世纪汉英中医辞典. 北京：人民军医出版社. 2004

17.　谢竹藩. 中医药常用名词术语英译. 北京：中国中医药出版社. 2004

18.　汪文娟. 汉英中医药词汇精要. 上海：上海科学技术文献出版社. 2004

19.　中医药学名词审定委员会. 中医药学名词. 北京：科学出版社. 2005

20.　欧明. 汉英中医词汇手册. 广州：广东科技出版社. 2005

21.　帅学忠. 汉英双解常用中医名词术语（再版）. 长沙：湖南科技出版社. 2006

22.　国家中医药管理局. 中医基础理论术语. 北京：中国标准出版社. 2006

23. 世界中医药学会联合会. 中医基本名词术语—中英对照国际标准. 北京: 人民卫生出版社. 2007

24. World Health Organization Western Pacific Region. *WHO International Standard Terminologies on Traditional Medicine in the Western Pacific Region.* Manila: Philippines. 2007

25. 李永安. 英汉西医—汉英中医常用词典. 北京: 北京理工大学出版社. 2010

26. 范波、黄莺. 英汉·汉英中医中药词汇手册. 上海: 上海外语教育出版社. 2012

27. 方廷钰、嵇波、吴青. 新汉英中医学词典（第2版）. 北京: 中国医药科技出版社. 2013

28. 杨明山. 精编常用中医英语字典. 上海: 复旦大学出版社. 2013

29. 梁晓春、孙华. 汉英中医学精要. 北京: 中国协和医科大学出版社. 2015

30. 李照国. 汉英双解中医临床标准术语辞典. 上海: 上海科技出版社. 2016

31. 谢竹藩. 新编汉英中医药分类词典（第二版）. 北京: 外文出版社. 2019

32. 方继良、崔永强. 简明汉英中医词汇手册. 广州: 广东科技出版社. 2019

33. 李照国、李汉平. 中医诊疗标准术语英译. 北京: 商务印书馆. 2020

34. 李永安、李亚军. 中医翻译二十讲. 西安: 西安交通大学出版社. 2021

35. World Health Organization. *WHO International Standard Terminologies on Traditional Chinese Medicine,* https://www.who.int/publications/i/item/9789240042322, accessed Oct. 20, 2023

# 中国历史年代简表 A Brief Chronology of Chinese History

| | | | |
|---|---|---|---|
| 远古时代 Prehistory | | | |
| 夏 Xia Dynasty | | | c. 2070 - 1600 BC |
| 商 Shang Dynasty | | | 1600 - 1046 BC |
| 周 Zhou Dynasty | 西周 Western Zhou Dynasty | | 1046 - 771 BC |
| | 东周 Eastern Zhou Dynasty<br>　春秋时代 Spring and Autumn Period<br>　战国时代 Warring States Period | | 770 - 256 BC<br>770 - 476 BC<br>475 - 221 BC |
| 秦 Qin Dynasty | | | 221 - 206 BC |
| 汉 Han Dynasty | 西汉 Western Han Dynasty | | 206 BC-AD 25 |
| | 东汉 Eastern Han Dynasty | | 25 - 220 |
| 三国 Three Kingdoms | 魏 Kingdom of Wei | | 220 - 265 |
| | 蜀 Kingdom of Shu | | 221 - 263 |
| | 吴 Kingdom of Wu | | 222 - 280 |
| 晋 Jin Dynasty | 西晋 Western Jin Dynasty | | 265 - 317 |
| | 东晋 Eastern Jin Dynasty<br>十六国 Sixteen States* | | 317 - 420<br>304 - 439 |
| 南北朝 Southern and Northern Dynasties | 南朝 Southern Dynasties | 宋 Song Dynasty | 420 - 479 |
| | | 齐 Qi Dynasty | 479 - 502 |
| | | 梁 Liang Dynasty | 502 - 557 |
| | | 陈 Chen Dynasty | 557 - 589 |
| | 北朝 Northern Dynasties | 北魏 Northern Wei Dynasty | 386 - 534 |
| | | 东魏 Eastern Wei Dynasty<br>北齐 Northern Qi Dynasty | 534 - 550<br>550 - 577 |
| | | 西魏 Western Wei Dynasty<br>北周 Northern Zhou Dynasty | 535 - 556<br>557 - 581 |

241

| 隋 Sui Dynasty | | 581 - 618 |
|---|---|---|
| 唐 Tang Dynasty | | 618 - 907 |
| 五代十国<br>Five Dynasties and Ten States | 后梁 Later Liang Dynasty | 907 - 923 |
| | 后唐 Later Tang Dynasty | 923 - 936 |
| | 后晋 Later Jin Dynasty | 936 - 947 |
| | 后汉 Later Han Dynasty | 947 - 950 |
| | 后周 Later Zhou Dynasty | 951 - 960 |
| | 十国 Ten States** | 902 - 979 |
| 宋 Song Dynasty | 北宋 Northern Song Dynasty | 960 - 1127 |
| | 南宋 Southern Song Dynasty | 1127 - 1279 |
| 辽 Liao Dynasty | | 907 - 1125 |
| 西夏 Western Xia Dynasty | | 1038 - 1227 |
| 金 Jin Dynasty | | 1115 - 1234 |
| 元 Yuan Dynasty | | 1206 - 1368 |
| 明 Ming Dynasty | | 1368 - 1644 |
| 清 Qing Dynasty | | 1616 - 1911 |
| 中华民国 Republic of China | | 1912 - 1949 |

### 中华人民共和国1949年10月1日成立
### People's Republic of China, founded on October 1, 1949

*"十六国"指东晋时期在我国北方等地建立的十六个地方割据政权，包括：汉（前赵）、成（成汉）、前凉、后赵（魏）、前燕、前秦、后燕、后秦、西秦、后凉、南凉、南燕、西凉、北凉、北燕、夏。

The "Sixteen States" refers to a series of local regimes established in the northern area and other regions of China during the Eastern Jin Dynasty, including Han (Former Zhao), Cheng (Cheng Han), Former Liang, Later Zhao (Wei), Former Yan, Former Qin, Later Yan, Later Qin, Western Qin, Later Liang, Southern Liang, Southern Yan, Western Liang, Northern Liang, Northern Yan, and Xia.

**"十国"指五代时期先后存在的十个地方割据政权，包括：吴、前蜀、吴越、楚、闽、南汉、荆南（南平）、后蜀、南唐、北汉。

The "Ten States" refers to the ten local regimes established during the Five Dynasties period, including Wu, Former Shu, Wuyue, Chu, Min, Southern Han, Jingnan (also Nanping), Later Shu, Southern Tang, and Northern Han.